Peripheral Nerve Disorders and Treatment

Edited by Hande Turker, Leonel Garcia Benavides, Guillermo Ramos Gallardo and Miriam Méndez Del Villar

Published in London, United Kingdom

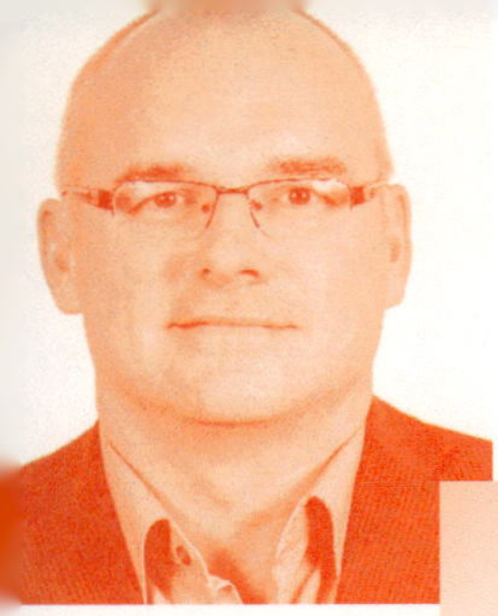
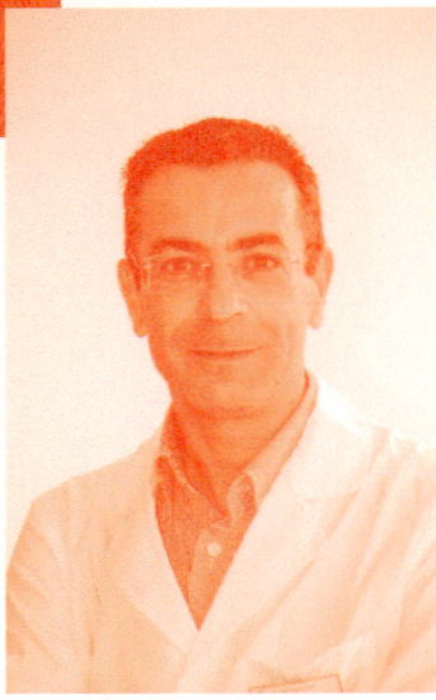
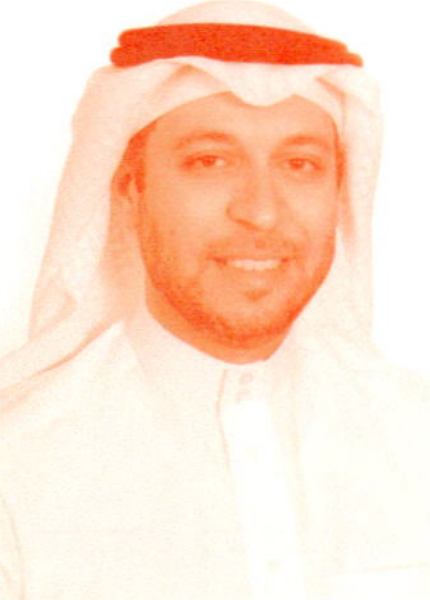
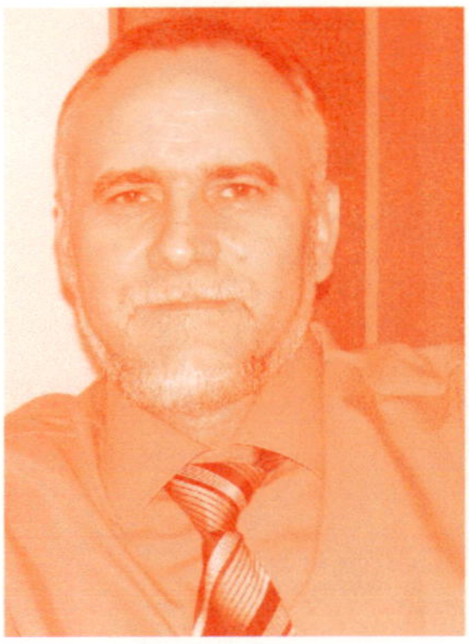
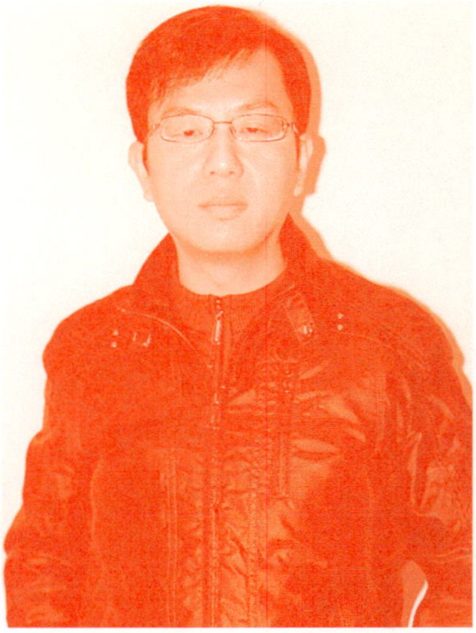
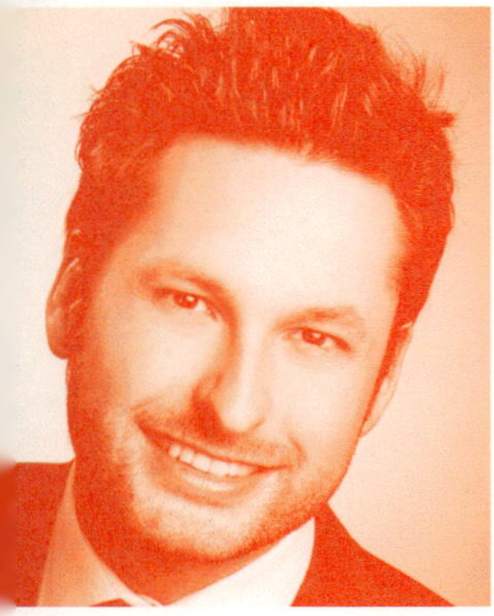
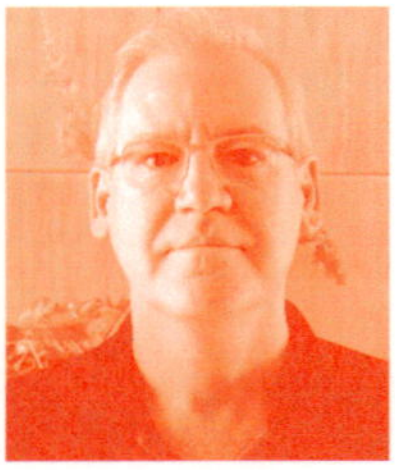

IntechOpen

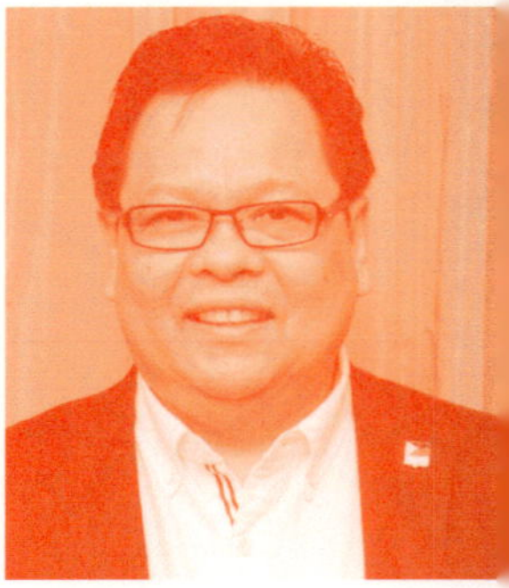
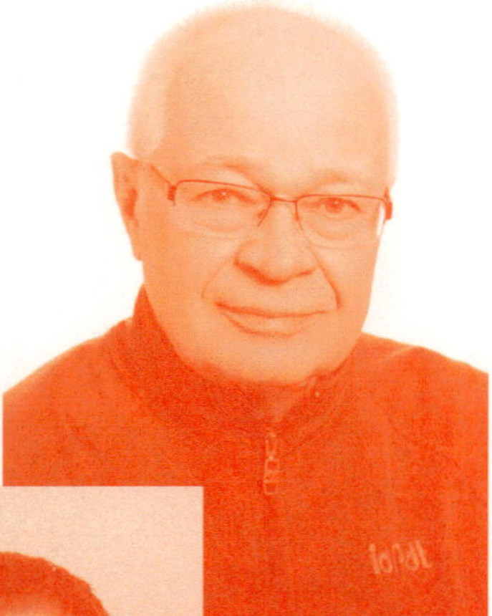
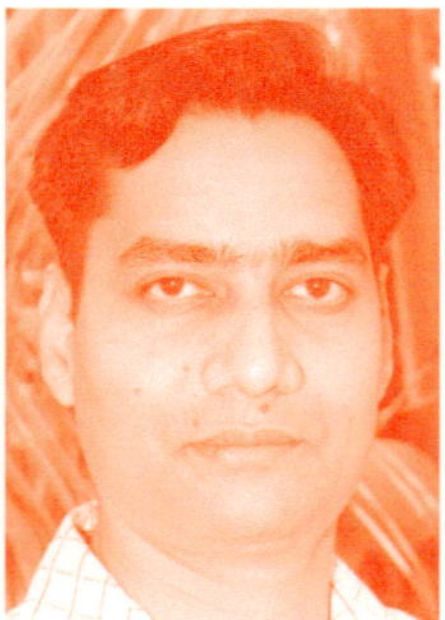
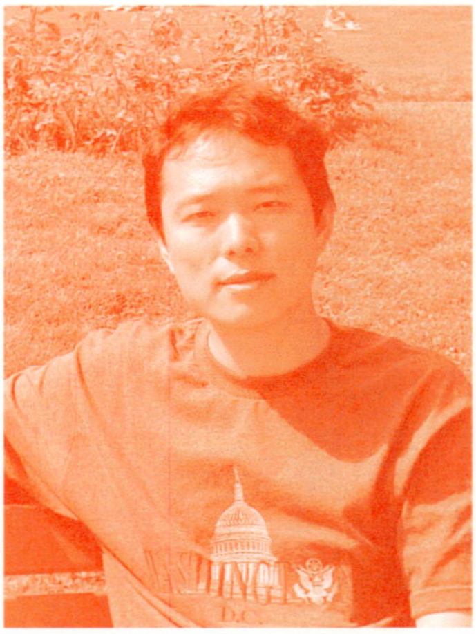
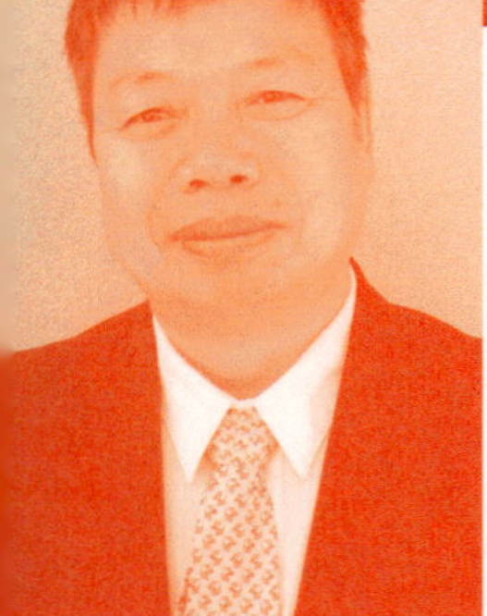
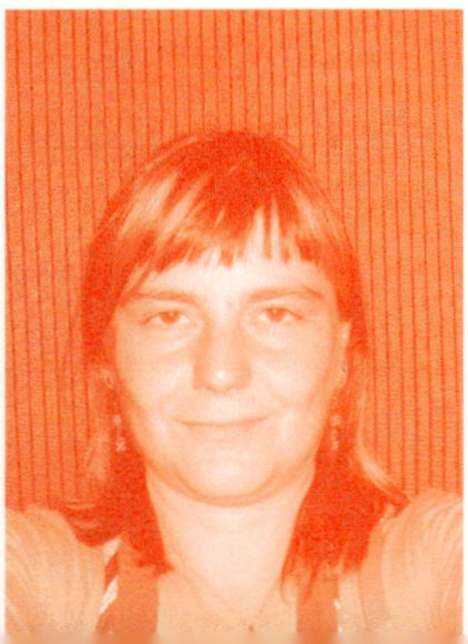

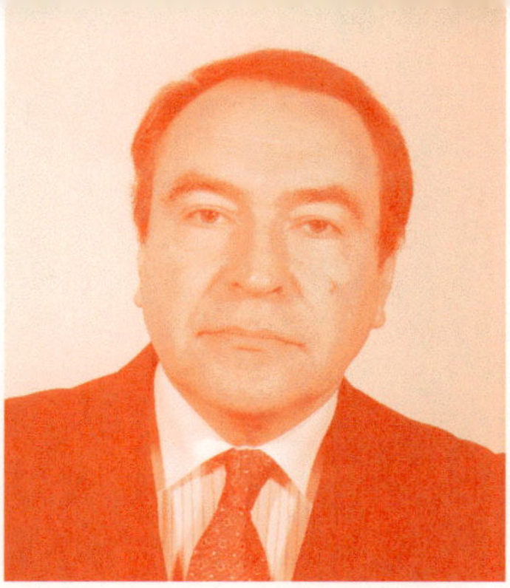
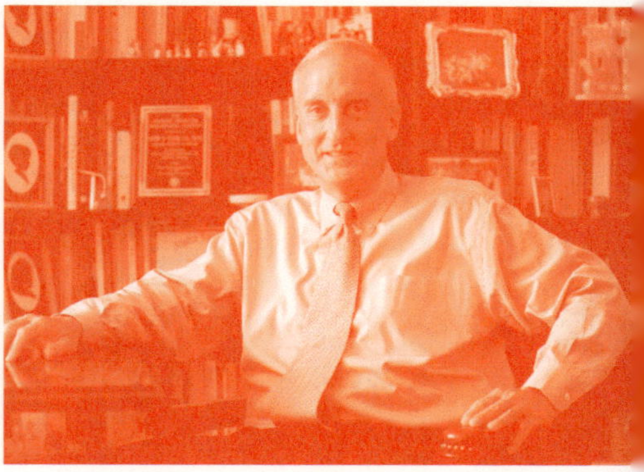
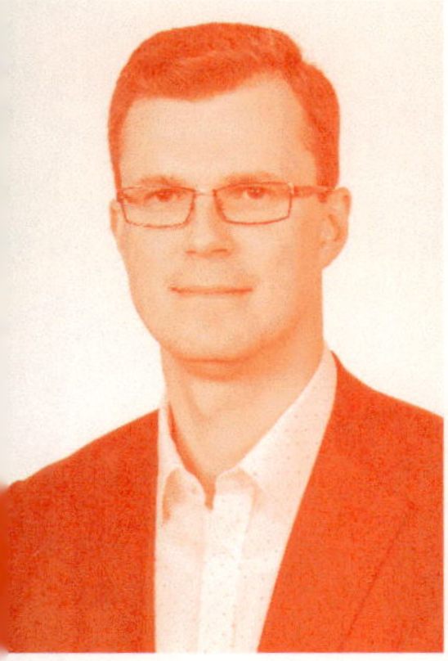
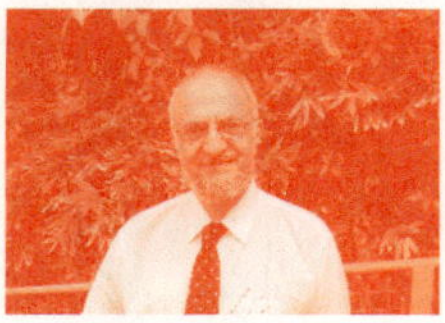
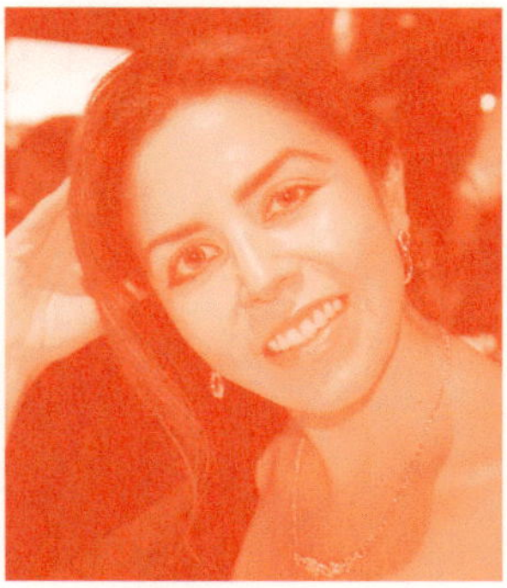

Supporting open minds since 2005

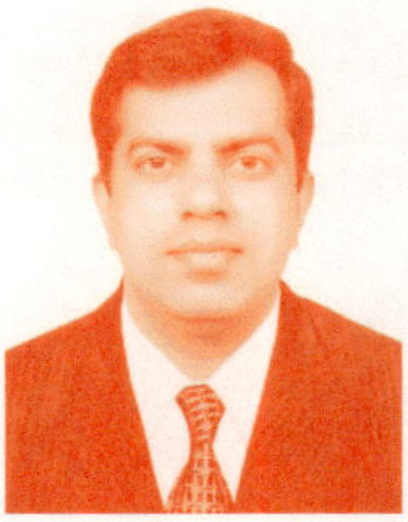
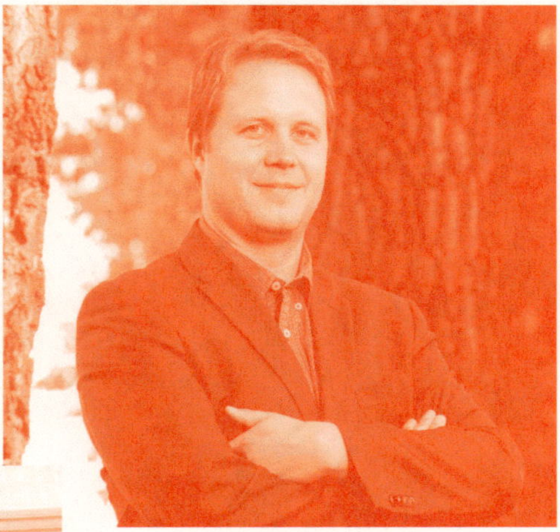
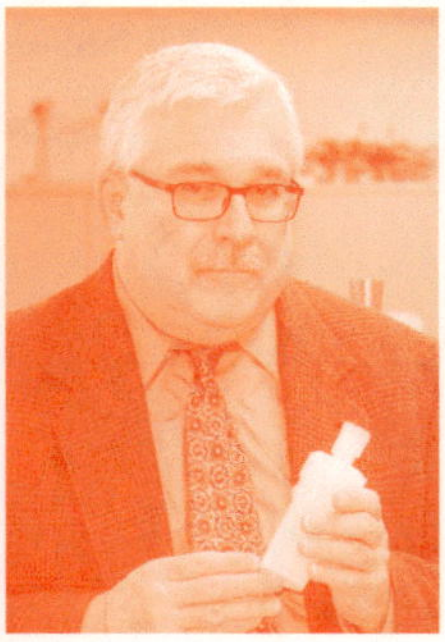
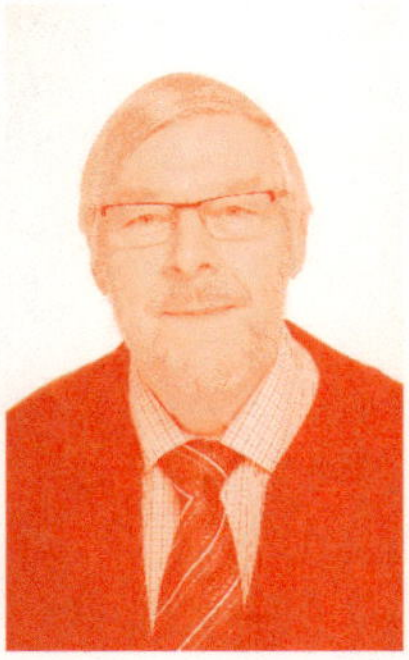
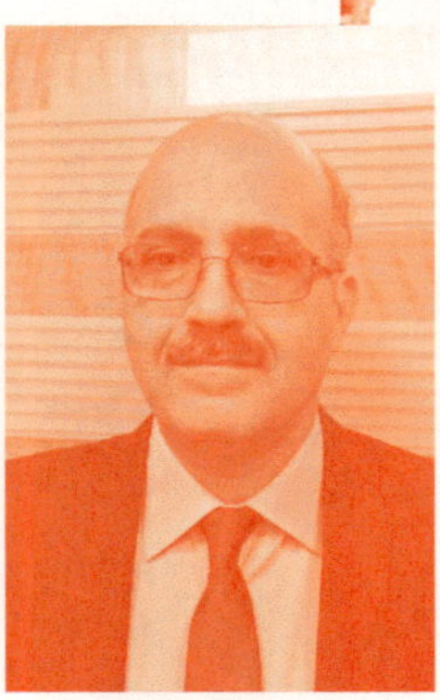
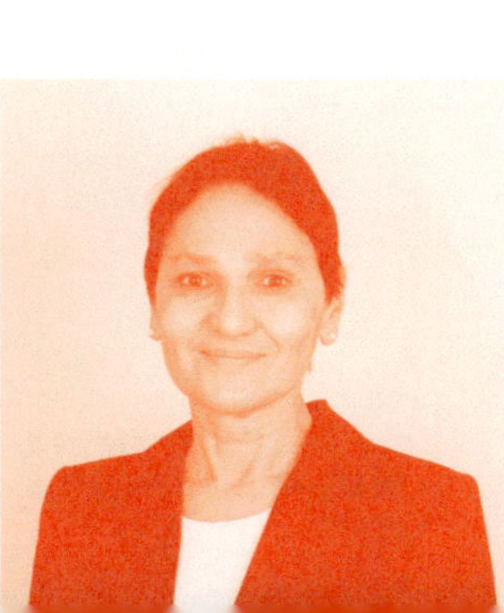
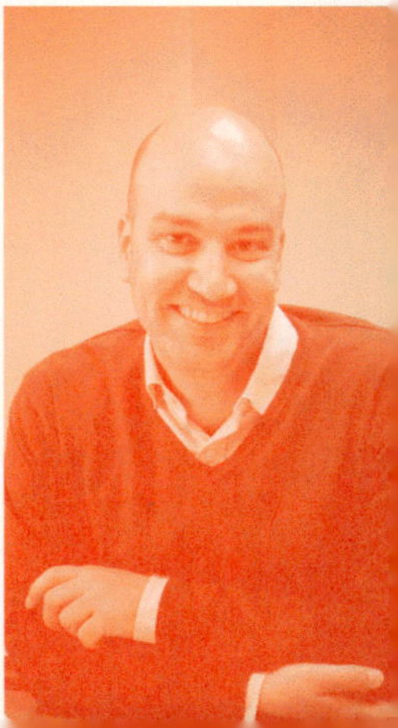

Peripheral Nerve Disorders and Treatment
http://dx.doi.org/10.5772/intechopen.78159
Edited by Hande Turker, Leonel Garcia Benavides, Guillermo Ramos Gallardo and Miriam Méndez Del Villar

Contributors
Chingcheng Huang, Hasan Md Arif Raihan, Poly Ghosh, Abhishek Biswas, Prasanna Lenka, Ameed Equbal, Vera Bril, Mohamed Bedewi, Daniele Coraci, Sherine Swify, Yashar Eshraghi, Maged Guirguis, Sarah J. Vitug, Leonel Garcia Benavides, Ana Colette Maurício, Mariana Vieira Branquinho, Rui Damásio Alvites, Rita Caseiro, Sílvia Santos Pedrosa, Ana Lúcia Luís, Stefano Geuna, Artur Varejão, Scott Ferris, Dong-Yuan Cao, Si-Qi Wei, Zhuo-Ying Tao, Yang Xue, Tayir Alon, Miriam Méndez del Villar, Leonel Garcia Valdés, Ming-Che Chiang

First published in London, United Kingdom, 2020 by IntechOpen
IntechOpen is the global imprint of INTECHOPEN LIMITED, registered in England and Wales, registration number: 11086078, 7th floor, 10 Lower Thames Street, London, EC3R 6AF, United Kingdom
Printed in Croatia

British Library Cataloguing-in-Publication Data
A catalogue record for this book is available from the British Library

Additional hard and PDF copies can be obtained from orders@intechopen.com

Peripheral Nerve Disorders and Treatment
Edited by Hande Turker, Leonel Garcia Benavides, Guillermo Ramos Gallardo and Miriam Méndez Del Villar
p. cm.
Print ISBN 978-1-78985-257-8
Online ISBN 978-1-78985-258-5
eBook (PDF) ISBN 978-1-83880-380-3

For EU product safety concerns:
IN TECH d.o.o., Prolaz Marije Krucifikse Kozulić 3, 51000 Rijeka, Croatia, info@intechopen.com or visit our website at intechopen.com.

Meet the editors

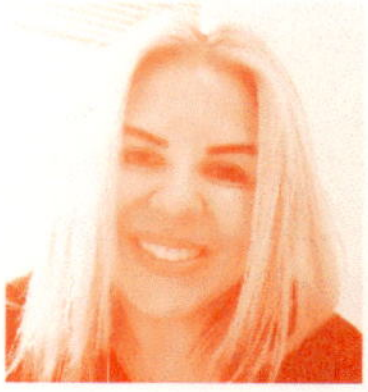

Hande Turker is a neurologist and clinical neurophysiologist. She has dealt with headache, neuropathic pain, neuromuscular diseases, dystonia, and electromyography and evoked potentials for nearly 30 years. She is the author of many publications, including several book chapters on evoked potentials and electromyography. Her main interests other than clinical neurophysiology are neuromuscular diseases with a special stress on neuropathies and neuropathic pain, headache, and botulinum toxin injections in movement disorders. She has been working at Ondokuz Mayıs University, Samsun, Turkey, since 2003. She is a professor of neurology and a lecturer, and teaches headache, neuropathic pain, neuromuscular diseases, and electromyography and evoked potentials at the same university, where she founded the "Evoked Potential Lab" and directed the EMG and EP Unit between 2003 and 2010. She is also the author of IntechOpen book chapters, including "Middle and long latency auditory evoked potentials and their usage in fibromyalgia and schizophrenia," "Neurological complications of hypothyroidism," and "Surface electromyography in sports and exercise." She is the editor of a number of IntechOpen books, including *Electrodiagnosis in New Frontiers of Clinical Research* and *Current Perspectives on Lesser-Known Aspects of Headache*. She has published more than 80 manuscripts, mostly original studies, speaks several foreign languages other than English, and is happily married.

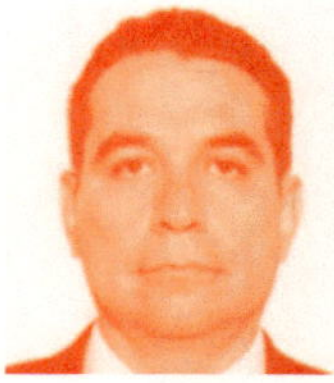

Leonel Garcia Benavides, MD and PhD, is a plastic and reconstructive surgeon, certificate number 940. He holds a PhD in Pharmacology from the University of Guadalajara, and is a member of the National Staff of Investigators, level 1. Dr. Benavides has been a research professor at the University of Guadalajara since 1987, is a member of the Clinical and Experimental Institute of the University of Guadalajara, and a member of the Staff of Specialists in the Plastic Surgery Department of the Civil Hospital of Guadalajara. He has experience in design, conduction, and analysis of clinical trials, is a coordinator of clinical investigation in the PhD program at the Health Sciences University Center of the University of Guadalajara, and has expertise in fibrogenesis and regeneration. Dr. Benavides is a member of AMCPER (Plastic and Reconstructive Surgery Mexican Association).

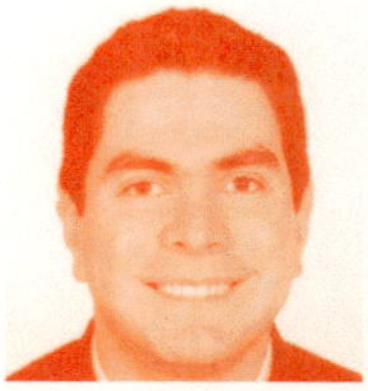

Dr. Guillermo Ramos Gallardo is a board-certified plastic surgeon specializing in facial, breast, and body reconstructive surgeries. He was trained at different hospitals in Mexico and the United States, with recognition from the Universidad Nacional Autonoma de Mexico, Universidad de Guadalajara, and University of Alabama at Birmingham. He is part of the staff at the Nuevo Hospital Civil de Guadalajara and he consults at the beautiful beach of Puerto Vallarta near the Pacific Ocean.

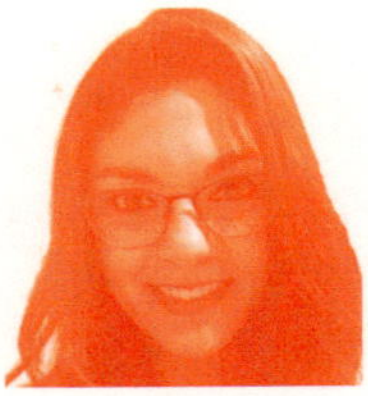

Miriam Méndez del Villar, PhD, is a professor and investigator at the University Center of Tonalá at the University of Guadalajara (Guadalajara, Jalisco, Mexico). She is Chief of the Department of Biomedical Sciences at the same university center. She is a nutritionist and obtained her PhD in Pharmacology in 2017; a year later she started her career as a teacher and researcher. She has published a total of 17 papers in the clinical research field, mainly related to cardiometabolic diseases. She participated as an investigator in 20 clinical trials, which has allowed her to be a member of the Mexican System of Investigators. Also, she has contributed to thesis direction of bachelor and PhD degree students, and has participated in the editing and writing of a number of books and book chapters.

Contents

Preface **XI**

Section 1
Mononeuropathies, Diagnosis and Treatment **1**

Chapter 1 **3**
Focal Upper Limb Mononeuropathies in Patients with Diabetes Mellitus
by Tayir Alon and Vera Bril

Chapter 2 **15**
Introductory Chapter: Current State of Carpal Tunnel Syndrome
by Leonel García Benavides, Miriam Méndez del Villar and Leonel Garcia Valdés

Chapter 3 **19**
Peripheral Nerve Imaging: Focus on Sonography
by Mohamed A. Bedewi, Daniele Coraci and Sherine Swify

Chapter 4 **31**
Orthotic Treatment Overview of Carpal Tunnel Syndrome
by Hasan Md Arif Raihan, Poly Ghosh, Prasanna Lenka, Ameed Equbal and Abhishek Biswas

Chapter 5 **49**
Biological and Preclinical Evaluations of Designed Optically Guided Medical Devices with Light Scattering Modules for Carpal Tunnel Syndrome Treatment and Surgical Procedure
by Ching-Cheng Huang and Ming-Che Chiang

Section 2
Peripheral Nerve Injury, Diagnosis and Treatment **65**

Chapter 6 **67**
Biomaterials and Cellular Systems at the Forefront of Peripheral Nerve Regeneration
by Rui Damásio Alvites, Mariana Vieira Branquinho, Ana Rita Caseiro, Sílvia Santos Pedrosa, Ana Lúcia Luís, Stefano Geuna, Artur Severo Proença Varejão and Ana Colette Maurício

Chapter 7 117
Risk and Reward: Avoiding Donor Morbidity and Maximizing Results in Nerve Transfer Surgery
by Scott Ferris

Section 3
New Insights For Neuropathic Pain 129

Chapter 8 131
Peripheral Sensitization
by Si-Qi Wei, Zhuo-Ying Tao, Yang Xue and Dong-Yuan Cao

Chapter 9 157
Interventional Treatment Options for Trigeminal Neuralgia
by Yashar Eshraghi, Sarah J. Vitug and Maged Guirguis

Preface

Neuropathies are intriguing subjects for clinicians, electromyographers, and peripheral nerve surgeons. The main reason for this assumption lies in the nature of these diseases, which still possess a number of secrets waiting to be discovered. This book contains current knowledge on neuropathies, which we believe you will find interesting. The subject of "neuropathies" comprises a number of topics, and each and every one could be the subject of a textbook.

This book was initially envisioned to solving problems in the diagnosis and therapy of neuropathies. The authors discuss the diagnosis and treatment of mononeuropathies, peripheral nerve injuries, and the new insights into the mechanisms of neuropathic pain. In some chapters of this book we also look at interesting and evocatory facts about interventional treatment options for neuropathic pain, which have "for" and "against" approaches.

This book should be read without prejudgment because the content may not be compatible with general but repeated assumptions and guidelines. However, I believe that this book may be an inspiration for many young investigators as well.

All in all, we have one major aim and that is to make you think deeply about neuropathies and neuropathic pain. We will be contented if we succeed.

Hande Turker
Ondokuz Mayis University,
Turkey

Leonel Garcia Benavides, Guillermo Ramos Gallardo and Miriam Méndez Del Villar
University of Guadalajara,
Mexico

Section 1

Mononeuropathies, Diagnosis and Treatment

Chapter 1

Focal Upper Limb Mononeuropathies in Patients with Diabetes Mellitus

Tayir Alon and Vera Bril

Abstract

In this chapter, we describe the prevalence, diagnostic methods, and treatment efficacy of compressive neuropathies of the median and the ulnar nerves in patients with diabetes mellitus (DM). Median neuropathy at the wrist is found in up to one-third of patients with DM, when demonstrated electrophysiologically, but is symptomatic as carpal tunnel syndrome (CTS) in a smaller proportion of these patients. It is clear that diabetes increases the risk of having clinical CTS. Diagnosis of CTS using nerve conduction studies is difficult in patients with DM and diabetic sensorimotor polyneuropathy (DSP) as median nerve conduction studies are affected predominantly by the diabetes state. We will discuss different electrodiagnostic and ultrasonography techniques for diagnosis and the outcomes of carpal tunnel release decompressive surgery in this special patient population. It is controversial whether DM is a risk factor for cubital tunnel syndrome or ulnar neuropathy at the elbow (UNE) or at the wrist (UNW). In this chapter, we will review the ultrasonographic and electrophysiological diagnostic techniques used in UNE and UNW and the efficacy of cubital tunnel release in DM patients.

Keywords: mononeuropathy, diabetes mellitus, carpal tunnel syndrome, nerve compression, diabetic sensorimotor polyneuropathy, median nerve, ulnar nerve, carpal tunnel syndrome, cubital tunnel syndrome

1. What causes the increased vulnerability to entrapment neuropathies in patients with DM

Entrapment neuropathies are more prevalent among patients with DM, and carpal tunnel syndrome (CTS) can guide a better understanding of the pathophysiology of entrapment neuropathies in this patient population. CTS is the most commonly studied entrapment syndrome and changes in the small arteries, such as vascular hypertrophy and intimal thickening, and noninflammatory fibroses of connective tissue are key pathologic features as discussed earlier in this book. In patients with DM, the reasons for the higher susceptibility to entrapment neuropathies are likely the combination of increased vulnerability of the nerves to compression arising from underlying diffuse DM-related nerve fiber injury and the presence of altered connective tissue structures within the carpal tunnel causing additional compression [1]. These two mechanisms are most likely relevant to all entrapment neuropathies in DM. Axonal, metabolic, and structural changes in DM that can lead to higher susceptibility to external injury are well-known. Less information on altered connective tissue structure in areas of nerve compression is available in this patient population. Deger et al. found a statistically significant increase in neoangiogenesis in subsynovial connective tissue in DM CTS cases, correlating with greater expression of vascular endothelial growth factor (VEGF), in subsynovial connective tissue in DM than what is present in CTS in patients without DM [2, 3]. These findings are consistent with the findings of Tekin et al., showing DM CTS patients, when compared with non-DM CTS patients, have higher rates of synovial edema and vascular proliferation and increased vascular wall thickness [4]. Thus the increased neovascularization, arising from a proposed ischemia-reperfusion mechanism, and more apparent in patients with DM, impinges the tissue compartment space within the carpal tunnel. In their recently published review, Sharma and Jaggi summarize the current knowledge regarding the role of transforming growth factor (TGF-β), VEGF, and interleukins in the subsynovial connective tissue in CTS patients, with and without diabetes [5].

2. Median compressive neuropathy at the wrist in patients with diabetes mellitus (DM)

The high prevalence of DM among patients with clinical CTS was first noted in 1962 by Blodgett et al. who reported DM in 59/915 or 6.4% of consecutive patients diagnosed with CTS [6]. A higher prevalence of DM among patients with CTS was described in 1972 by Phalen, who reported DM in 14.6% or in 56/384 consecutive patients diagnosed with CTS [7]. Subsequent studies demonstrated a similar prevalence with the calculated odds ratio (OR) of 3.02 for CTS in DM [8, 9]. The risk of CTS is further increased in DM patients with neuropathic symptoms, as shown by Perkins et al., who found a similar frequency of clinical CTS in 14% of nonneuropathic DM subjects, increasing to 30% in those with diabetic sensorimotor polyneuropathy (DSP) of varying severity [10]. This prospective cohort study evaluated clinical CTS, defined rigorously, across a broad spectrum of DSP patients (**Table 1**). Pourmemari and Shiri performed a meta-analysis including over 90,000 subjects and examined DM as a risk factor for CTS. They found the association to be more modest with an unadjusted OR estimate of about 2 and less when controlling for potential confounding factors with a pooled estimate OR was 1.59 [11, 12]. This outcome may be related to varying definitions of CTS within different studies included in the meta-analysis.

Comi et al. examined the prevalence of median neuropathy in patients with DM using electrophysiological studies, but not symptoms and signs of CTS.

Paresthesiae in hands or marked preponderance of sensory symptoms in the hands
Nocturnal hand symptoms awakening the patient
Symptoms precipitated by activities such as holding a newspaper or driving a car and relieved by hand shaking
Predilection for radial digits
Weak thenar muscles
Upper limb sensory loss solely within the distribution of the median nerve
4/6 criteria required to diagnose CTS in those with DM with or without DSP [10] *Electrodiagnostic criteria for CTS unreliable in the presence of DM [10]*

Table 1.
Clinical criteria for the diagnosis of carpal tunnel syndrome in diabetes patients.

11.2% showed electrophysiology indicating focal median neuropathy. The prevalence was higher (16.1%) among patients with DSP [13]. Other studies have shown even higher rates, up to 23%, of asymptomatic median compressive neuropathy at the wrist in patients with DM [14]. The issue with this approach is that CTS is a clinical diagnosis, and the Perkins study showed that electrophysiological changes at the carpal tunnel are related to DSP and not indicative of the presence of CTS [10]. All of these studies indicate that although median neuropathy at the wrist is relatively common in patients with DM when tested by nerve conduction studies, clinical CTS is not found in a similar proportion. Symptomatic CTS was described in 9% of DM subjects in an early study [15], and the lifetime risk of symptomatic CTS in type 1 diabetes was calculated more recently to be as high as 85% by Singh et al. [16].

2.1 Electrophysiologic and ultrasonographic diagnostic techniques used in median compressive neuropathy at the wrist in patients with DM

DSP symptoms might mimic those of CTS in clinical practice. Nonetheless, clear symptoms for a diagnosis of CTS can be established even in those with advanced DSP [10]. Establishing the diagnosis of CTS based solely on electrophysiological diagnostic criteria is unreliable in DM patients, since the changes in electrophysiological parameters are due to DSP rather than CTS [10]. Various electrophysiological parameters are thought to distinguish CTS from DSP in subjects with DM, but none were found to be different in those with and without CTS in a population of subjects with DM [10]. Parameters such as median nerve distal motor or sensory latency, comparison of ratios of median (ulnar latencies or amplitudes or sensory conduction velocities), and others failed to differentiate those patients who had clinical CTS from those who did not in subjects with DM [10]. Consequently, in subjects with DM, it is prudent to be cautious in attributing changes in electrophysiological parameters to CTS rather than DM with or without DSP.

There have been attempts to establish electrodiagnostic methods that might distinguish CTS from DSP but doubt about the results which arise from the Perkins study [10]. For example, the median nerve distal motor latency or the median nerve sensory distal onset latency when stimulating at the palm or at the wrist crease has been reported to show differences between DM patients with CTS and idiopathic CTS in a small study [17], but those same parameters were not reliable in larger studies [10, 18]. Additional studies have reported other parameters that may be useful in diagnosis such as the median-radial sensory latency difference from the thumb, which showed 94% sensitivity in one study [19], and for a cutoff of 0.55, 82% sensitivity and 80% specificity in another study [18]. As the ulnar nerve is also susceptible to entrapment, a comparison of median nerve parameters to radial nerve parameters was thought to be preferable. Other studies have suggested using the median-ulnar sensory latency difference measured from the ring finger with 86% sensitivity in one study [19], and for a cutoff of 0.35, 90% sensitivity and 85% specificity in another study [18], although this sensory latency difference could not identify those with CTS in a larger study [10]. The lumbrical-interosseous latency difference was significantly different between CTS patients with and without DM, with sensitivity of up to 88.4% in two studies [17, 20], and for a cutoff of 1 ms had 78% sensitivity in another study [21].

Small studies have examined the feasibility of using ultrasonography to distinguish CTS with DM cases from DSP alone. Kim et al. found that all the cross-sectional areas (CSA) of the median nerve were larger in DSP patients compared with healthy controls, and the CSA of the median nerve at the wrist revealed no significant differences among DSP patients with and without CTS; however, patients with CTS (with and without DM) had larger CSAs at the wrist and a higher wrist/forearm ratio compared with DSP patients. The cutoff value for the CSA at the wrist that yielded the highest sensitivity and specificity was 11.6 mm [22]. A smaller study found no ultrasound measurement (distal median CSA, wrist-forearm ratio, wrist-forearm difference) reached significance to detect CTS in patients with DSP [17].

2.2 Treatment efficacy for CTS in patients with DM

The outcome of open decompression of the median nerve by sectioning the carpal transverse ligament in DM patients has been evaluated in many studies. Several studies, with a post-procedure follow-up of up to 2 years, showed similar beneficial outcomes, in nerve conduction studies and symptoms, for patients with and without DM [23–29]. Some studies found that electrodiagnostic findings and assessment of symptoms and clinical signs improved significantly in both DM patients and in non-DM patients but that the improvement was less in the diabetic group [30–33]. Zhang et al. demonstrated an association of DM with an increased risk for secondary surgery following carpal tunnel decompression. They tested a total of 904 patients with and without DM, for a median follow-up length of less than a year [34]. Gulabi et al. compared the symptomatic outcome at 6 months and 10 years after decompression of 27 patients with DM and 42 patients with idiopathic CTS. They found that at 6 months, the outcomes were similar for the DM and non-DM groups, but at 10 years the DM group had poor outcomes possibly due to progression of DSP in the DM group [35]. Recently published results of a randomized controlled prospective study comparing the outcome of endoscopic carpal tunnel release versus open carpal tunnel release in DM patients suggest that the endoscopic approach is more beneficial for patients with diabetes. In this study, the patients who underwent endoscopic carpal tunnel release had better relief of symptoms and better function scores, less pillar pain and tenderness at 12 weeks after surgery, faster regain of grip and pinching functions, significantly faster return to work and significant improvement in wound healing, as well as reduction in wound infection and complications [36].

The evidence to date indicates that surgery in DM patients with CTS leads to an improvement in symptoms and signs of CTS that is very similar to non-DM patients with CTS. Given this background, it is reasonable to offer surgical therapy to DM patients with CTS when conservative treatments have failed, as is the case for idiopathic CTS, i.e., in those without DM.

3. Compressive ulnar neuropathy at the elbow in patients with DM

There is controversy over whether or not cubital tunnel syndrome is more common in those with DM. Stamboulis et al. found 12.2% of patients with cubital tunnel syndrome had DM [37]. In other studies, the prevalence of DM was the same in patients with cubital tunnel syndrome as in the general population, i.e., 6% in both groups, when the diagnosis of cubital tunnel syndrome was established on the combination of symptoms, objective clinical findings, and electrodiagnostic tests [38], and the severity of symptoms was also similar between those with and without DM [39]. In a case-control study, including only patients who had undergone ulnar nerve decompression, DM was not found to be a risk factor for ulnar neuropathy at the elbow [40]. The question of whether DM is a risk factor for cubital tunnel syndrome remains uncertain.

3.1 Electrophysiologic and ultrasonographic diagnostic techniques used in compressive ulnar neuropathy at the elbow in patients with DM

Rota et al. tested DM patients for ulnar neuropathy at the elbow irrespective of clinical symptoms and found that 34% had electrodiagnostic features of ulnar dysfunction due to chronic compression at the elbow. Most of the patients with neurophysiological abnormalities were asymptomatic, and only 6% had sensory symptoms and showed clinical signs of cubital tunnel syndrome [41].

It has been demonstrated in large cohorts that sensory nerve conduction velocity and amplitudes of sensory nerve action potentials are markedly lower in DM patients than in healthy controls, even more so in DM patients with known DSP [38, 42–45]. As asymptomatic ulnar nerve entrapment at the elbow (UNE) is relatively common among patients with DM, possibly due to the underlying DSP similar to CTS, when the diagnosis of cubital tunnel syndrome in patients with DM with or without DSP is in question, we rely mainly on changes in the motor conduction electrophysiologic parameters. Schady et al. studied 20 DM patients with cubital tunnel syndrome, demonstrated by hand wasting and weakness. All patients also had signs of DSP in the lower limbs. The nerve conduction studies in this cohort showed markedly reduced ulnar nerve compound muscle action potential (CMAP) amplitudes with a mean value of 1.2 versus 7.4 mV in controls and also reduced ulnar/median CMAP amplitude ratios. Less sensitive than the CMAP amplitudes was the ulnar nerve motor conduction velocity. This was disproportionately slowed across the elbow segment in only 8 of 34 affected ulnar nerves [43].

Only two studies have used ultrasonography for the diagnosis of ulnar compressive neuropathy at the elbow in patients with DM. Kang et al. had demonstrated that the cross-sectional area (CSA) of the ulnar nerve at the cubital tunnel outlet was significantly greater in patients with DSP than in healthy controls, with no correlation to nerve conduction study results [46]. It is possible that the larger CSA is a marker of DM and not specific for DSP or of ulnar compressive neuropathy at the elbow in patients with DM, as might be inferred from the second study. Chen et al. tested DM patients with and without confirmed DSP. They found that CSA of the ulnar nerve at the cubital tunnel outlet was greater in DM patients than that in the healthy control group, yet no difference was detected in the CSA of the ulnar nerve between DM patient with and without DSP [47]. These studies found no correlation between the cubital tunnel syndrome and the CSA or even between asymptomatic UNE and the CSA.

3.2 Treatment efficacy for ulnar compressive neuropathy at the elbow in patients with DM

A recent US national database review of more than 15,000 patients who underwent ulnar nerve decompression at the cubital tunnel found a low incidence of failure of cubital tunnel release requiring ipsilateral revision, but the presence of DM was an independent risk factor for revision with an adjusted odds ratio of 1.27 [48]. The presence of DM did not increase the risk for infection following cubital tunnel release [49]. Other smaller studies have found that DM is not associated with a poor surgical result, either clinically or electrophysiologically [50], or with a greater likelihood of revision surgery [51–53]. When satisfaction with treatment was assessed, having DM was not associated with a higher likelihood of dissatisfaction with treatment [54].

4. Ulnar compressive neuropathy at the wrist in patients with diabetes mellitus (DM)

Ulnar entrapment at the wrist is far less common, and thus less studied, than ulnar nerve entrapment at the elbow. The prevalence of DM among patients with ulnar tunnel syndrome at the wrist is yet to be determined, as no large-scale study has assessed the presence of this potential entrapment. In fact, the only relevant data comes from a single retrospective study of 31 patients who had an ulnar nerve palsy treated by ulnar tunnel (Guyon's canal) release, and 6 patients or 19% had DM [55].

4.1 Electrophysiologic and ultrasonographic diagnostic techniques used in ulnar compressive neuropathy at the wrist in patients with DM

The diagnosis of ulnar tunnel syndrome at the wrist is routinely based on the motor nerve conduction study parameters. Rota et al. tested DM patients for ulnar neuropathy at the wrist, and their electrodiagnostic study demonstrated relevant neurophysiological abnormalities in 11% of the patients, all of whom had DSP as well. The paper does not state how many of the patients presenting with these electrophysiological abnormalities were symptomatic [41].

There is a single paper regarding the use of ultrasonography for the diagnosis of ulnar compressive neuropathy at the wrist in patients with DM. Chen et al., who tested DM patients with and without confirmed DSP, showed that the CSA of the ulnar nerve at Guyon's canal was greater in DM patients than in the healthy control group, yet no difference was detected in the CSA of ulnar nerves between DM patients with and without DSP. No potential relationship to clinical signs or symptoms of ulnar tunnel syndrome was examined in this study [47].

5. Summary

Upper limb mononeuropathies are common in patients with DM with the most common being CTS. The diagnosis of CTS in DM is a clinical diagnosis as the electrophysiologic and ultrasonographic parameters do not reliably distinguish between CTS and DSP. Treatment can be highly effective in CTS patients with DM whether or not DSP is present. Asymptomatic ulnar nerve electrophysiological abnormalities are common in DM, but it is unclear if clinical entrapment syndromes at the elbow are more common or not. The success of surgical decompression of the ulnar nerve at the elbow in those with DM is similar to that in non-DM patients. Ulnar nerve entrapment at the wrist is infrequent, and data on diagnosis and treatment is limited or unavailable.

Acknowledgements

No funding was received for preparation of this manuscript.

Conflict of interest

All authors declare that they have no conflict of interest pertinent to this work.

Author details

Tayir Alon[1] and Vera Bril[2,3]*

1 Edith Wolfson Medical Center, Holon, Israel

2 Ellen and Martin Prosserman Centre for Neuromuscular Diseases, Division of Neurology, Department of Medicine, University Health Network, University of Toronto, Toronto, Canada

3 Institute for Research and Medical Consultations, Imam Abdulrahman Bin Faisal University, Dammam, Saudi Arabia

*Address all correspondence to: vera.bril@utoronto.ca

References

[1] Dyck PJ, Giannini C. Pathologic alterations in the diabetic neuropathies of humans. Journal of Neuropathology and Experimental Neurology. 1996;**55**(12):1181-1193. Available from: https://academic.oup.com/jnen/article-lookup/doi/10.1097/00005072-199612000-00001

[2] Deger AN, Deger H, Taser F. The role of neoangiogenesis and vascular endothelial growth factor in the development of carpal tunnel syndrome in patients with diabetes. Nigerian Journal of Clinical Practice. 2016;**19**(2):189-195. Available from: http://www.ncbi.nlm.nih.gov/pubmed/26856279

[3] Taser F, Deger AN, Deger H. Comparative histopathologic evaluation of diabetic, hypothyroid and idiopathic carpal tunnel syndrome. Turkish Neurosurgery. 2016;**27**(6):991-997. Available from: http://www.ncbi.nlm.nih.gov/pubmed/27651338

[4] Tekin F, Sürmeli M, Şimşek H, Ceran C, Tezcan S, Taner ÖF, et al. Comparison of the histopathological findings of patients with diabetic and idiopathic carpal tunnel syndrome. International Orthopaedics. 2015;**39**(12):2395-2401. Available from: http://link.springer.com/10.1007/s00264-015-2790-y

[5] Sharma D, Jaggi AS, Bali A. Clinical evidence and mechanisms of growth factors in idiopathic and diabetes-induced carpal tunnel syndrome. European Journal of Pharmacology. 2018;**837**:156-163. Available from: http://www.ncbi.nlm.nih.gov/pubmed/30125568

[6] Blodgett RC, Lipscomb PR, Hill RW. Incidence of hematologie disease in patients with carpal tunnel syndrome. Journal of the American Medical Association. 1962;**182**(7):814-815. Available from: http://jama.jamanetwork.com/article.aspx?doi=10.1001/jama.1962.03050460106017a

[7] Phalen GS. The carpal-tunnel syndrome. Clinical evaluation of 598 hands. Clinical Orthopaedics and Related Research. 1972;**83**:29-40. Available from: http://www.ncbi.nlm.nih.gov/pubmed/5014825

[8] Karpitskaya Y, Novak CB, Mackinnon SE. Prevalence of smoking, obesity, diabetes mellitus, and thyroid disease in patients with carpal tunnel syndrome. Annals of Plastic Surgery. 2002;**48**(3):269-273. Available from: http://www.ncbi.nlm.nih.gov/pubmed/11862031

[9] Eversmann WW, Ritsick JA. Intraoperative changes in motor nerve conduction latency in carpal tunnel syndrome. The Journal of Hand Surgery. 1978;**3**(1):77-81. Available from: http://linkinghub.elsevier.com/retrieve/pii/S0363502378801191

[10] Perkins BA, Olaleye D, Bril V. Carpal tunnel syndrome in patients with diabetic polyneuropathy. Diabetes Care. 2002;**25**(3):565-569. Available from: http://www.ncbi.nlm.nih.gov/pubmed/11874948

[11] Pourmemari MH, Shiri R. Diabetes as a risk factor for carpal tunnel syndrome: A systematic review and meta-analysis. Diabetic Medicine. 2016;**33**(1):10-16. DOI: 10.1111/dme.12855

[12] Geoghegan JM, Clark DI, Bainbridge LC, Smith C, Hubbard R. Risk factors in carpal tunnel syndrome. The Journal of Hand Surgery. 2004;**29**(4):315-320. Available from: http://journals.sagepub.com/doi/10.1016/J.JHSB.2004.02.009

[13] Comi G, Lozza L, Galardi G, Ghilardi MF, Medaglini S, Canal N. Presence of carpal tunnel syndrome in diabetics: Effect of age, sex, diabetes duration and polyneuropathy. Acta Diabetologica Latina. 1985;**22**(3):259-262. Available from: https://link.springer.com/content/pdf/10.1007%2FBF02590778.pdf

[14] Albers JW, Brown MB, Sima AAF, Greene DA. Frequency of median mononeuropathy in patients with mild diabetic neuropathy in the early diabetes intervention trial (EDIT). Muscle and Nerve. 1996;**19**(2):140-146. Available from: http://www.ncbi.nlm.nih.gov/pubmed/8874414

[15] Mulder DW, Lambert EH, Bastron JA, Sprague RG. The neuropathies associated with diabetes mellitus. A clinical and electromyographic study of 103 unselected diabetic patients. Neurology. 1961;**11**(4 Pt 1):275-284. Available from: http://www.ncbi.nlm.nih.gov/pubmed/13773672

[16] Singh R, Gamble G, Cundy T. Lifetime risk of symptomatic carpal tunnel syndrome in type 1 diabetes. Diabetic Medicine. 2005;**22**(5):625-630. DOI: 10.1111/j.1464-5491.2005.01487.x

[17] Hassan A, Leep Hunderfund AN, Watson J, Boon AJ, Sorenson EJ. Median nerve ultrasound in diabetic peripheral neuropathy with and without carpal tunnel syndrome. Muscle and Nerve. 2013;**47**(3):437-439. DOI: 10.1002/mus.23677

[18] Gazioglu S, Boz C, Cakmak VA. Electrodiagnosis of carpal tunnel syndrome in patients with diabetic polyneuropathy. Clinical Neurophysiology. 2011;**122**(7):1463-1469. Available from: https://ac.els-cdn.com/S1388245711000137/1-s2.0-S1388245711000137-main.pdf?_tid=455fa08c-ce76-11e7-a88e-00000aacb362&acdnat=1511239482_ed527fcb50dc5e024b4a4b1ea89ad6ee

[19] Imada M, Misawa S, Sawai S, Tamura N, Kanai K, Sakurai K, et al. Median-radial sensory nerve comparative studies in the detection of median neuropathy at the wrist in diabetic patients. Clinical Neurophysiology. 2007;**118**(6):1405-1409. Available from: https://ac.els-cdn.com/S1388245707000946/1-s2.0-S1388245707000946-main.pdf?_tid=496688fa-ce79-11e7-85fb-00000aacb362&acdnat=1511240786_8144071cb3dc9ec9e4c72c8d4003dd59

[20] Yagci I, Gunduz OH, Sancak S, Agirman M, Mesci E, Akyuz G. Comparative electrophysiological techniques in the diagnosis of carpal tunnel syndrome in patients with diabetic polyneuropathy. Diabetes Research and Clinical Practice. 2010;**88**(2):157-163. Available from: https://ac.els-cdn.com/S0168822710000872/1-s2.0-S0168822710000872-main.pdf?_tid=84d8434e-ce77-11e7-95a9-00000aacb361&acdnat=1511240018_2b24f72b235788bf9cf0425a9e54c009

[21] Vogt T, Mika A, Thömke F, Hopf HC. Evaluation of carpal tunnel syndrome in patients with polyneuropathy. Muscle & Nerve. 1997;**20**(2):153-157. Available from: http://www.ncbi.nlm.nih.gov/pubmed/9040652

[22] Kim L-N, Kwon H-K, Moon H-I, Pyun S-B, Lee H-J. Sonography of the median nerve in carpal tunnel syndrome with diabetic neuropathy. American Journal of Physical Medicine & Rehabilitation. 2014;**93**(10):897-907. Available from: http://content.wkhealth.com/linkback/openurl?sid=WKPTLP:landingpage&an=00002060-201410000-00007

[23] Thomsen NOB, Cederlund R, Rosén I, Björk J, Dahlin LB. Clinical outcomes of surgical release among diabetic patients with carpal tunnel syndrome: Prospective follow-up with matched

controls. The Journal of Hand Surgery. 2009;**34**(7):1177-1187. Available from: http://linkinghub.elsevier.com/retrieve/pii/S0363502309003451

[24] Mondelli M, Padua L, Reale F, Signorini AM, Romano C. Outcome of surgical release among diabetics with carpal tunnel syndrome. Archives of Physical Medicine and Rehabilitation. 2004;**85**(1):7-13. Available from: http://www.archives-pmr.org/article/S0003-9993(03)00770-6/pdf

[25] Thomsen NOB, Rosén I, Dahlin LB. Neurophysiologic recovery after carpal tunnel release in diabetic patients. Clinical Neurophysiology. 2010;**121**(9):1569-1573. Available from: http://linkinghub.elsevier.com/retrieve/pii/S1388245710003020

[26] Jenkins PJ, Duckworth AD, Watts AC, McEachan JE. The outcome of carpal tunnel decompression in patients with diabetes mellitus. Journal of Bone and Joint Surgery. 2012;**9494**(6):811-814. Available from: http://bjj.boneandjoint.org.uk/content/jbjsbr/94-B/6/811.full.pdf

[27] Zyluk A, Puchalski P. A comparison of outcomes of carpal tunnel release in diabetic and non-diabetic patients. Journal of Hand Surgery. 2013;**38**(5):485-488. Available from: http://journals.sagepub.com/doi/10.1177/1753193412469781

[28] Ozer K, Malay S, Toker S, Chung KC. Minimal clinically important difference of carpal tunnel release in diabetic and nondiabetic patients. Plastic and Reconstructive Surgery. 2013;**131**(6):1279-1285. Available from: http://content.wkhealth.com/linkback/openurl?sid=WKPTLP:landingpage&an=00006534-201306000-00008

[29] Watchmaker JD, Watchmaker GP. Independent variables affecting outcome of carpal tunnel release surgery. The Hand. 2018;**13**(3):285-291. Available from: http://journals.sagepub.com/doi/10.1177/1558944717703739

[30] Ozkul Y, Sabuncu T, Kocabey Y, Nazligul Y. Outcomes of carpal tunnel release in diabetic and non-diabetic patients. Acta Neurologica Scandinavica. 2002;**106**(3):168-172. Available from: http://www.ncbi.nlm.nih.gov/pubmed/12174177

[31] Isik C, Uslu M, Inanmaz ME, Karabekmez FE, Kose KC. The effects of diabetes on symptoms of carpal tunnel syndrome treated with mini-open surgery. Acta Orthopaedica Belgica. 2013;**79**(4):381-385. Available from: http://www.ncbi.nlm.nih.gov/pubmed/24205766

[32] Haupt WF, Wintzer G, Schop A, Löttgen J, Pawlik G. Long-term results of carpal tunnel decompression. Assessment of 60 cases. Journal of Hand Surgery. 1993;**18**(4):471-474. Available from: http://www.ncbi.nlm.nih.gov/pubmed/8409659

[33] Yucel H. Factors affecting symptoms and functionality of patients with carpal tunnel syndrome: A retrospective study. Journal of Physical Therapy Science. 2015;**27**(4):1097-1101. Available from: https://www.jstage.jst.go.jp/article/jpts/27/4/27_jpts-2014-727/_pdf

[34] Zhang D, Blazar P, Earp BE. Rates of complications and secondary surgeries of mini-open carpal tunnel release. The Hand. 2018:155894471876522. Available from: http://journals.sagepub.com/doi/10.1177/1558944718765226

[35] Gulabi D, Cecen G, Guclu B, Cecen A. Carpal tunnel release in patients with diabetes result in poorer outcome in long-term study. European Journal of Orthopaedic Surgery and Traumatology. 2014;**24**(7):1181-1184. Available from: http://link.springer.com/10.1007/s00590-014-1418-z

[36] Ismail M, Schuh A, Ibrahim M. Outcome of Endoscopic Carpal Tunnel Release Versus Open Carpal Tunnel Release in Diabetic Patients: A Randomized Controlled Prospective Double Blinded Study. 2018. Available from: http://www.oatext.com/pdf/GMT-1-108.pdf [Accessed: 27 September 2018]

[37] Stamboulis E, Vassilopoulos D, Kalfakis N. Symptomatic focal mononeuropathies in diabetic patients: Increased or not? Journal of Neurology. 2005;**252**(4):448-452. Available from: http://link.springer.com/10.1007/s00415-005-0672-8

[38] Mondelli M, Aretini A, Rossi S. Ulnar neuropathy at the elbow in diabetes. American Journal of Physical Medicine & Rehabilitation. 2009;**88**(4):278-285. Available from: http://content.wkhealth.com/linkback/openurl?sid=WKPTLP:landingpage&an=00002060-200904000-00006

[39] Naran S, Imbriglia JE, Bilonick RA, Taieb A, Wollstein R. A demographic analysis of cubital tunnel syndrome. Annals of Plastic Surgery. 2010;**64**(2):177-179. Available from: http://content.wkhealth.com/linkback/openurl?sid=WKPTLP:landingpage&an=00000637-201002000-00016

[40] Bartels RHMA, Verbeek ALM. Risk factors for ulnar nerve compression at the elbow: A case control study. Acta Neurochirurgica. 2007;**149**(7):669-674. Discussion 674. Available from: http://link.springer.com/10.1007/s00701-007-1166-5

[41] Rota E, Zavaroni D, Parietti L, Iafelice I, De Mitri P, Terlizzi E, et al. Ulnar entrapment neuropathy in patients with type 2 diabetes mellitus: An electrodiagnostic study. Diabetes Research and Clinical Practice. 2014;**104**(1):73-78. Available from: https://www.sciencedirect.com/science/article/pii/S0168822714000540

[42] Zhang Y, Li J, Wang T, Wang J. Amplitude of sensory nerve action potential in early stage diabetic peripheral neuropathy: An analysis of 500 cases. Neural Regeneration Research. 2014;**9**(14):1389-1394. Available from: http://www.ncbi.nlm.nih.gov/pubmed/25221597

[43] Schady W, Abuaisha B, Boulton AJM. Observations on severe ulnar neuropathy in diabetes. Journal of Diabetes and its Complications. 2017;**12**(3):128-132. Available from: https://ac.els-cdn.com/S1056872797000949/1-s2.0-S1056872797000949-main.pdf?_tid=69558916-c9b2-11e7-b816-00000aacb362&acdnat=1510715557_4d8fa0a0aab177eeab422e8a99981877

[44] Rota E, Quadri R, Fanti E, Isoardo G, Poglio F, Tavella A, et al. Electrophysiological findings of peripheral neuropathy in newly diagnosed type II diabetes mellitus. Journal of the Peripheral Nervous System. 2005;**10**(4):348-353. DOI: 10.1111/j.1085-9489.2005.00046.x

[45] Jang JE, Kim YT, Park BK, Cheong IY, Kim DH. Subclinical ulnar neuropathy at the elbow in diabetic patients. Annals of Rehabilitation Medicine. 2014;**38**(1):64-71. Available from: https://synapse.koreamed.org/DOIx.php?id=10.5535/arm.2014.38.1.64

[46] Kang S, Kim SH, Yang SN, Yoon JS. Sonographic features of peripheral nerves at multiple sites in patients with diabetic polyneuropathy. Journal of Diabetes and its Complications. 2016;**30**(3):518-523. Available from: https://ac.els-cdn.com/S1056872715004900/1-s2.0-S1056872715004900-main.pdf?_tid=1eb9bf84-c959-11e7-82af-00000aab0f6b&acdnat=1510677206_8d523dc6437dc142dedade48e77373c7

[47] Chen J, Wang C-L, Wu S, He S, Ren J. The feasibility of using

high-resolution ultrasonography to assess ulnar nerve in patients with diabetes mellitus. Journal of Ultrasonography. 2017;**17**:160-166. Available from: http://jultrason.pl/uploads/dm_artykuly/jou-2017-0024.pdf

[48] Camp CL, Ryan CB, Degen RM, Dines JS, Altchek DW, Werner BC. Risk factors for revision surgery following isolated ulnar nerve release at the cubital tunnel: A study of 25,977 cases. Journal of Shoulder and Elbow Surgery. 2017;**26**(4):710-715. Available from: http://linkinghub.elsevier.com/retrieve/pii/S1058274616305730

[49] Camp CL, Tebo CC, Degen RM, Dines JS, Altchek DW, Werner BC. Patient-related risk factors for infection following ulnar nerve release at the cubital tunnel: An analysis of 15,188 cases. Orthopaedic Journal of Sports Medicine. 2018;**6**(5). Available from: http://www.pearldiverinc.com

[50] Friedman RJ, Cochran TP. A clinical and electrophysiological investigation of anterior transposition for ulnar neuropathy at the elbow. Archives of Orthopaedic and Trauma Surgery. 1987;**106**(6):375-380. Available from: http://www.ncbi.nlm.nih.gov/pubmed/3435238

[51] Krogue JD, Aleem AW, Osei DA, Goldfarb CA, Calfee RP. Predictors of surgical revision after in situ decompression of the ulnar nerve. Journal of Shoulder and Elbow Surgery. 2015;**24**(4):634-639. Available from: https://www.sciencedirect.com/science/article/pii/S105827461400682X

[52] Gaspar MP, Kane PM, Putthiwara D, Jacoby SM, Osterman AL. Predicting revision following in situ ulnar nerve decompression for patients with idiopathic cubital tunnel syndrome. The Journal of Hand Surgery. 2016;**41**(3):427-435. Available from: http://linkinghub.elsevier.com/retrieve/pii/S0363502315015889

[53] Gaspar MP, Jacoby SM, Osterman AL, Kane PM. Risk factors predicting revision surgery after medial epicondylectomy for primary cubital tunnel syndrome. Journal of Shoulder and Elbow Surgery. 2016;**25**(4):681-687. Available from: https://www.sciencedirect.com/science/article/pii/S1058274615005959

[54] Roh YH, Kim S, Gong HS, Baek GH. Clinical features affecting the patient-based outcome after minimal medial epicondylectomy for cubital tunnel syndrome. Journal of Plastic, Reconstructive & Aesthetic Surgery. 2018. Available from: https://www.sciencedirect.com/science/article/pii/S174868151830192X

[55] Murata K, Shih JT, Tsai TM. Causes of ulnar tunnel syndrome: A retrospective study of 31 subjects. The Journal of Hand Surgery. 2003;**28**(4):647-651. Available from: https://ac.els-cdn.com/S0363502303001473/1-s2.0-S0363502303001473-main.pdf?_tid=5f7bde2c-c9ad-11e7-8e60-00000aab0f01&acdnat=1510713393_4d6ab2b3c461d4f88fc3ee4bc6b97c1f

Chapter 2

Introductory Chapter: Current State of Carpal Tunnel Syndrome

Leonel García Benavides, Miriam Méndez del Villar and Leonel Garcia Valdés

1. General considerations

The carpal tunnel is a fibrous extension that connects the anterior compartment of the forearm with the palm of the hand. It is delimited by the pisiform bone medially, by the hamate bone laterally, and the base of the scaphoid and trapezoid bone and the roof by the dorsal radiocarpal ligaments of the carpus. Through the carpal tunnel, various anatomical structures pass, such as the median nerve (NM), the nine flexor tendons of the fingers and the thumb, the nerve is located on a superficial plane over the tendons and medial to the radio palmar artery, although its trajectory and division has numerous anatomical variant, which present with a frequency of 11% approximately in general population. The principal anatomical variants are the presence of a residual median artery (5% of the population) and the anastomosis of Martin-Gruber, a motor communication between the median and cubital nerves at the forearm, present in 5–10% of the population [1].

The American Association of Orthopedic Surgery (AAOS) defines carpal tunnel syndrome as the most common mononeuropathy [2]. It has a prevalence of 3.8% in general population, and has an incidence of 276 for every 100,000 citizens [3, 4]. It affects women in major proportions than men, and 50–60% of all patients have bilateral affection [5].

CTS can be divided into primary or idiopathic, which is associated with repetitive manual activity and secondary, which is associated to other pathologies.

Other studies have established that idiopathic CTS is caused by a spaced conflict between the limits of the tunnel and the content that passes through it, which increases the pressure inside the tunnel and consequently alters the blood flow to the MN, provoking an inflammatory response and epineural edema. In healthy individuals, the pressure inside the tunnel (with the hand at neutral position) varies from 3 to 5 mm/hg. However, in patients with CTS, this pressure in the same conditions is an average of 35 mmHg [6].

Other studies have encountered morphological changes in the synovial tissue that surrounds the tendons. The principal findings have been inflammation, edema and fibrosis [7]. Multiple biochemical changes in the proteoglycans have also been reported, which causes a decrease in the capacity of the tendon to deform and compress itself [6, 7].

These findings suggest that the changes in the tendons and the synovial tissues caused by repetitive manual activity and aging degeneration, increase the volume of content inside the tunnel, resulting in the compression of the MN, leading eventually to CTS [8]. Another suggested mechanism of lesion is through repetitive microtrauma of the MN caused by alterations on the kinetic movement of the tendon and the nerve [7].

The pathologies with a higher prevalence associated to CTS are diabetes mellitus; with a prevalence of 14–30% of the patients, in which a dysfunction of The Schwann cells, alterations of the immune system and microangiopathy have been associated. Pregnancy is associated to diverse alterations of the peripheral nervous system. Amyloidosis through a direct lesion to the MN by amyloid deposits [5]. This book describes not only the prevalence, but also diagnostic methods and treatment efficacy of compressive neuropathies of the median and the ulnar nerves in patients with diabetes mellitus.

The clinical manifestations can be classified into three stages according its severity: first stage: nocturnal paresthesia and pain in the carpal region [3]. The sensorial symptoms and the pain continue through the day and the sensation of a having clumsy hand is added, presenting difficulties to perform precise activities with the hand. Atrophy of the thenar eminence and weakness are present in the final stage [4].

It is common that the patients mention the necessity to shake the hand to try to diminish the symptoms, which is known as Flick's sign [9], which reflects the presence of abnormalities in nerve conduction studies; it has a sensibility and specificity of 93 and 96%, respectively. Due to the variety in the clinical manifestations, we should focus on the new evaluation instruments used with the intent of identifying symptomatology and evolution, such as the Boston questionnaire [10, 11].

Provocative tests are numerous maneuvers that exist to detect CTS, these include Phalen's test, which has a sensibility of 57–91% and a specificity of 33.86%; Reversed Phalen's test, which has a sensibility of 23–60% and a specificity of 64–87%; Tinel's Sign, which has a sensibility of 67% and a specificity of 55–87% and Durkan's Test; which has a sensibility of 64% and a specificity of 83% [12, 13].

To quantitatively establish the electrophysiological state of the nerve and select the definitive treatment, it is required to perform nerve conduction studies, which have a sensibility and specificity of 85 and 94%, respectively, and are realized comparing the findings of the MN to another nerve [2, 14].

2. New approaches to be followed

This book will approach the current treatment regarding CTS, which can be classified into surgical and non-surgical. The decision of which treatment to follow is difficult and the severity of the symptoms must be taken into consideration. In patients with moderate to severe manifestations, surgical treatment must be considered as the first choice. Non-surgical treatment includes different therapeutic actions such as steroid injections or use of drugs with antioxidant and anti-inflammatory properties. Splinting is recommended before any option of treatment; surgical or non-surgical; the proper application of orthotic splinting is analyzed as well in this book as a special chapter to show the clinical convenience of a novel light guided medical device.

Author details

Leonel García Benavides[1,2]*, Miriam Méndez del Villar[1] and Leonel Garcia Valdés[2]

1 Division of Health Sciences, Cutonala, University of Guadalajara, Jalisco, México

2 Hospital Civil de Guadalajara "Fray Antonio Alcalde", Guadalajara, Jalisco, México

*Address all correspondence to: drleonelgb@hotmail.com

References

[1] Herrera E, Anaya C, Abril AM, Lozano Wilson M, Avellaneda YC, Cruz AM. Anastomosis Martin-Gruber: Aspectos anatómicos y electrofisiológicos. Revista de la Universidad Industrial de Santander. Salud. 2009;**41**(2):157-168. Available from: http://www.scielo.org.co/scielo.php?script=sci_arttext&pid=S0121 08072009000200007&lng=en [Accessed: 01 June 2019]

[2] American Academy of Ortopedic Surgeons. Clinical Practice Guidelines on Diagnosis of Carpal Tunnel Syndrome. 1st ed. Rosemont, Illinois: American Academy of Orthopedic Surgeons; 2007. p. 5

[3] Mondelli M, Giannini F, Giacchi M. Carpal tunnel syndrome incidence in a general population. Neurology. 2002;**58**(2):289-294

[4] Bland JD, Rudolfer SM. Clinical surveillance of carpal tunnel syndrome in two areas of the United Kingdom, 1991-2001. Journal of Neurology, Neurosurgery, and Psychiatry. 2003;**74**(12):1674-1679

[5] Le Blanc K, Cestia W. Carpal tunnel syndrome. American Family Physician. 2011;**83**(8):952-958

[6] Werner R, Armstrong T. Carpal tunnel syndrome: Ergonomic risk factors and intracarpal canal pressure, carpal tunnel syndrome. Physical Medicine and Rehabilitation Clinics of North America. 1997;**8**:555-569

[7] Copplieters MW, Alshami AM. Longitudinal excursion and strain in the median nerveduring novel nerve gliding exercises for carpal tunnel syndrome. Journal of Orthopaedic Research. 2007;**25**:972-980

[8] Rojviroj S, Sirichativapee W, Kowsuwon W, Wongwiwat-tananon J, Tamnanthong N, Jeeravipoolvarn P. Pressures in the carpal tunnel. A comparison between patients with carpal tunnel syndrome and normal subjects. Journal of Bone and Joint Surgery. British Volume (London). 1990;**72**:516-518

[9] Pryse-Phillips WE. Validation of a diagnostic sign in carpal tunnel syndrome. Journal of Neurology, Neurosurgery, and Psychiatry. 1984;**47**(8):870-872. DOI: 10.1136/jnnp.47.8.870

[10] Levine DW, Simmons BP, Koris MJ, Daltroy LH, Hohl GG, Fossel AH, et al. A self-administered questionnaire for the assessment of severity of symptoms and functional status in carpal tunnel syndrome. The Journal of Bone and Joint Surgery. American Volume. 1993;**75**(11):1585-1592

[11] Miyamoto Meirelles L, Gomes dos santos JB, Leonel dos santos LL, Branco MA, Faloppa F, Mattioli Leite V, Fernandes CH. Evaluation of Boston questionnaire applied at late postoperative period of carpal tunnel syndrome operated with the Paine retinaculatome through palmar port. Acta Ortopédica Brasileira. 2006;**14**(3):126-132

[12] D'Arcy CA, McGee S. Does this patient have carpal tunnel syndrome? Journal of the American Medical Association. 2000;**283**(23):3110-3117. DOI: 10.1001/jama.283.23.3110

[13] Mac Dermid JC, Wessel J. Clinical diagnosis of carpal tunnel syndrome: A systematic review. Journal of Hand Therapy. 2004;**17**:309-319. DOI: 10.1197/j.jht.2004.02.015

[14] de Jesus Filho AG, do Nascimento BF, Amorim Mde C, Naus RA, Loures Ede A, Moratelli L. Comparative study between physical examination, electroneuromyography and ultrasonography in diagnosing carpal tunnel syndrome. Revista Brasileira de Ortopedia. 2014;**49**(5):446-451. DOI: 10.1016/j.rboe.2014.09.002

Chapter 3

Peripheral Nerve Imaging: Focus on Sonography

Mohamed A. Bedewi, Daniele Coraci and Sherine Swify

Abstract

The diagnosis of different peripheral nerve disorders is basically established by electrodiagnostic tests; the assessment of the function of peripheral nerve disorders is estimated by nerve conduction tests (NCT) and electromyography (EMG). The need for more information about nerve morphology mandated the usage of more diagnostic tools. This role is now achieved by means of peripheral nerve imaging consisting mainly of magnetic resonance imaging (MRI) and ultrasonography. In this chapter we will clarify the role of imaging in the diagnosis of peripheral nerve disorders, concentrating more on the role of modern high-resolution ultrasound, considering its advantages like cheap price, dynamic ability, and possibility of comparison with the contralateral side at the same setting.

Keywords: peripheral, ultrasound, imaging, peripheral nerves

1. Introduction

Diseases of the peripheral nerves are common in the setting of clinical practice. The traditional way of the diagnosis of peripheral nerve disorders is made by neurophysiology and clinical assessment. These tools give information about the functional status of the involved nerve, the presence of nerve damage, and the degree of demyelination [1]; however, the need for more information about nerve morphology mandated the usage of more diagnostic tools. This role is now enhanced by means of peripheral nerve imaging consisting mainly of magnetic resonance imaging (MRI) and ultrasonography, with special ability to assess small-sized and difficult nerves [2].

2. Magnetic resonance imaging

Magnetic resonance imaging is a noninvasive imaging technique that has the ability to differentiate pathological peripheral nerves from healthy ones. MRI is also useful in the demonstration of the topographic anatomy of the peripheral nerves. MRI uses a strong magnetic field to create a net magnetization in the involved tissues, then disruption of this magnetization with pulse, and change of direction resulting in T1- and T2-weighted images. Basic MRI study of the peripheral nerves uses T2-weighted images (with fat suppression) detecting the site of injury as sharp hyperintense (as a result of local edema), in comparison to the nearby healthy nerves which appear as isointense. As nerve regeneration resumes, the degree of hyperintensity will gradually return to isointesntiy. Fat suppression is used for better visualization. Typically a 1.5 Tesla machine is used, with better results if a stronger magnet is utilized (3 Tesla). As a result of research, a newer MRI technique was developed, which is diffuse tensor imaging (DTI), tracking the diffusion of water molecules, depending on the fact that there is a difference in diffusion pattern between the healthy and injured nerves. The healthy nerves appear as linear structures which maintain diffusion in an anisotropic pattern restricting the movement linearly. If there is structural damage, the water molecules diffuse in an orthogonal pattern [3–5]. Among the disadvantages of MRI are the high-cost and long examination time. Also MRI is not tolerated by claustrophobic patients, and the examination is not suitable for patients with pacemakers and many types of surgical implants.

3. Ultrasound

The first report of nerve ultrasound was by Bruno Fornage in the year 1988, who used a linear transducer with a 5–7.5 MHZ frequency. Ultrasound is a cheap modality, which allows examination of the whole nerve at the same setting, plus the contralateral side [2]. This modality is also dynamic, with excellent spatial resolution and nonionizing radiation and good patient compliance. Among the disadvantages of ultrasound is that the procedure is operator dependent, limited ability to visualize deep nerves and long learning curve [3]. Initially ultrasound was mainly used to assess the cross-sectional area (CSA). Among the additional parameters assessed by peripheral nerve ultrasound is the so called "nerve density," representing hypoechoic/hyperechoic ratio [6]. The use extended field of view is sometimes needed.

4. Ultrasound exam and findings

In order to perform an accurate examination, a good knowledge of the anatomical landmark of each nerve is essential. A linear high-frequency transducer 5–18 MHZ (**Figure 1**) is used for ultrasound examination. Another transducer (Hockey stick) is occasionally referred to (**Figure 2**). Peripheral nerves should be imaged in both short and long axes; they appear in short axis as hypoechoic structures with peculiar fascicular pattern "honeycomb appearance." We recommend beginning the examination in short-axis scan, as differentiation of the nerves is difficult from the surrounding longitudinally oriented structures like tendons.

Topographic anatomy is always helpful in identifying specific nerves. The probe position must be placed perpendicular to scanned nerve in order to avoid anisotropy phenomenon. The simplest measurement of nerve caliber is made by estimating the cross-sectional area (CSA). Two known methods are used for this purpose, the older of which is the ellipse technique, and the newer and most recommended one is the tracer method, by which the nerve is measured inside the hyperechoic epineurium. Each nerve has a reference value, which when exceeded is a sign of disease. Loss of the fascicular pattern could be a sign of disease, as a result of edema/congestion. The cause is variable, the most important of which is compression neuropathy. Other types of neuropathies also exist like immune-mediated neuropathies. The role of ultrasound in traumatic injuries is quiet important. The most important issue in trauma is to make sure of nerve continuity, and if there is an injury, it is complete or partial [7–12]. New techniques like three-dimensional imaging and compound imaging were developed during the last 10 years. Measurement of stiffness of the nerve is established by elastography [6].

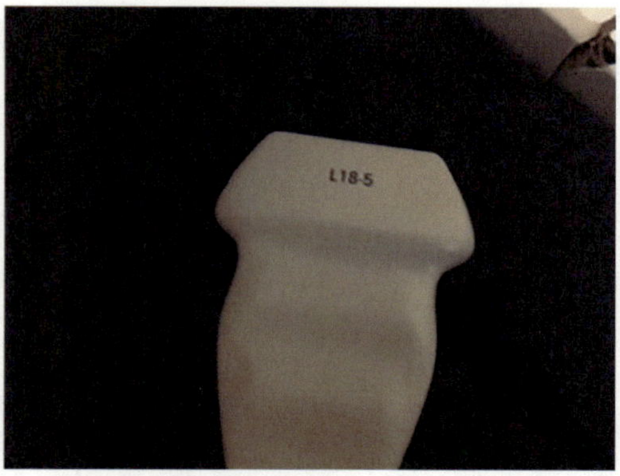

Figure 1.
Linear transducer.

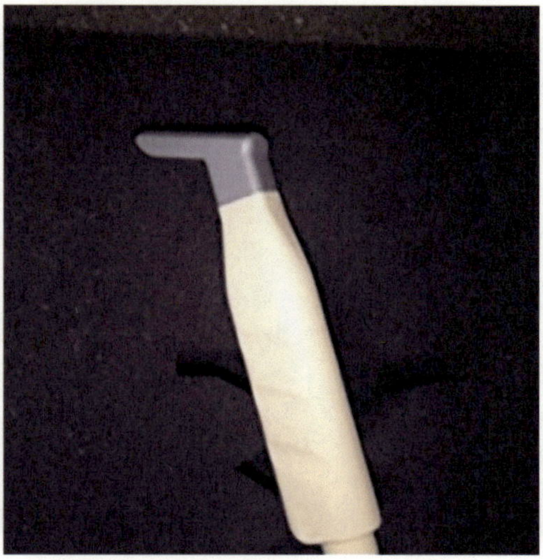

Figure 2.
Hockey stick transducer.

5. Brachial plexus

The brachial plexus consists of the network of nerves providing the sensorimotor supply of the upper limb (C5-T1) (**Figure 3**) [6]. Brachial plexus injuries are common in different types of trauma, including car accidents and falls, which could lead to severe impairment. Some lesions are minor, and patients could recover without surgery. The presence of a good diagnostic tool is essential in this manner [13]. Brachial plexus lesions are common, whether traumatic or nontraumatic. Traumatic lesions could also be open or closed.

6. Upper limb nerves

The radial nerve arises from the C5–C8 nerve roots. This nerve has a peculiar spiral course around the humerus, maintaining direct contact with the humerus, making the nerve highly sustainable to trauma (**Figure 4**). At the distal upper arm, the radial nerve divides into superficial (mainly sensory) and deep (mainly motor) branches (**Figure 5**). The ulnar nerve (**Figure 6**) arises from C8-T1nerve roots.

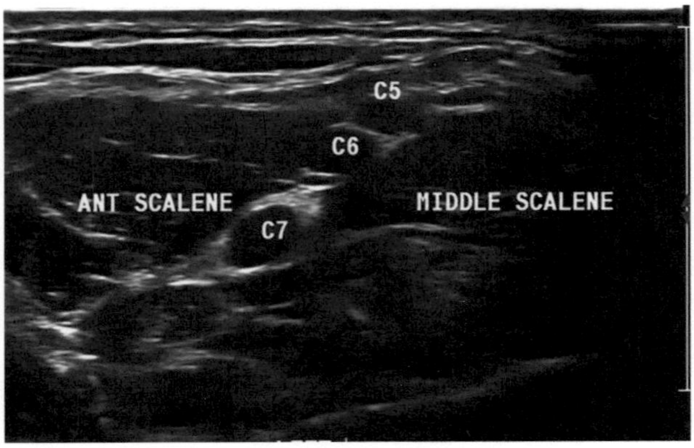

Figure 3.
Short-axis scan of the C5, C6, and C7 nerve roots, in the interscalene groove, between the middle scalene and anterior scalene muscles. s, scalene muscle.

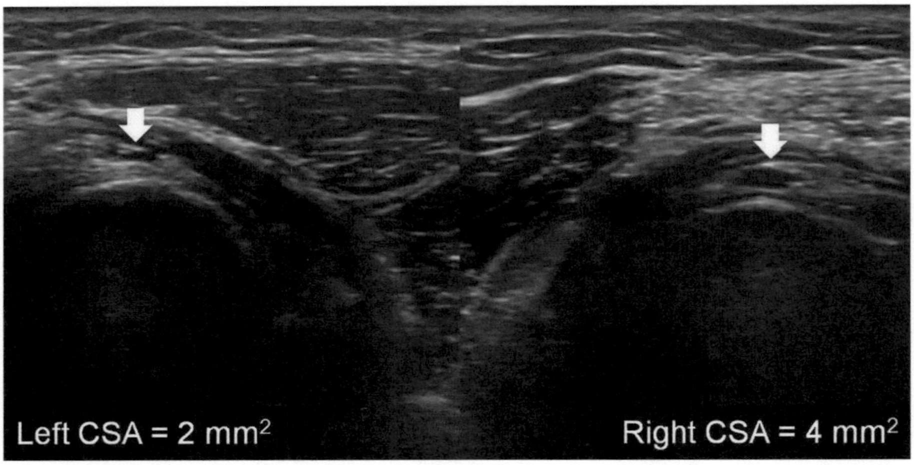

Figure 4.
A case of upper limb trauma with humeral bone fracture and following deficit in finger extension. The posterior interosseous nerve is larger than the contralateral side.

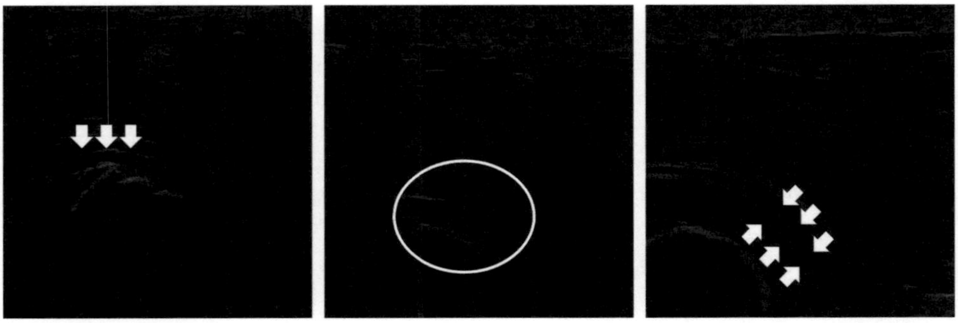

Figure 5.
A case of blade trauma in the forearm. The patient presents with plegia of the extensor digitorum communis muscle. From right to left, the images show the posterior interosseous nerve course from proximal to distal. In the image at the center, the nerve is not visible (ellipse), while proximally (right) and distally (left), the nerve is depictable (arrows).

Two common levels of injury/entrapment to the ulnar nerve are the cubital tunnel (**Figure 7**) at the level of the medial epicondyle of the elbow joint (which represents

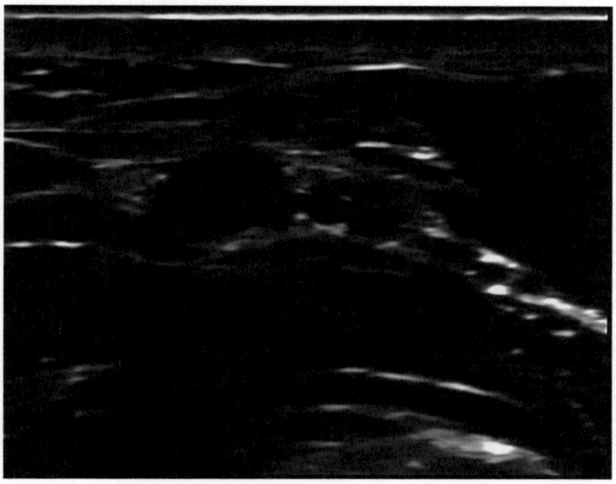

Figure 6.
Short-axis scan of the ulnar nerve at the forearm.

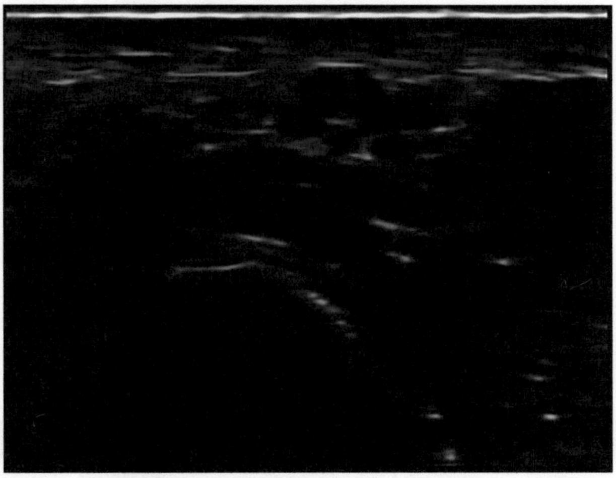

Figure 7.
Short-axis scan of the ulnar nerve at the cubital tunnel.

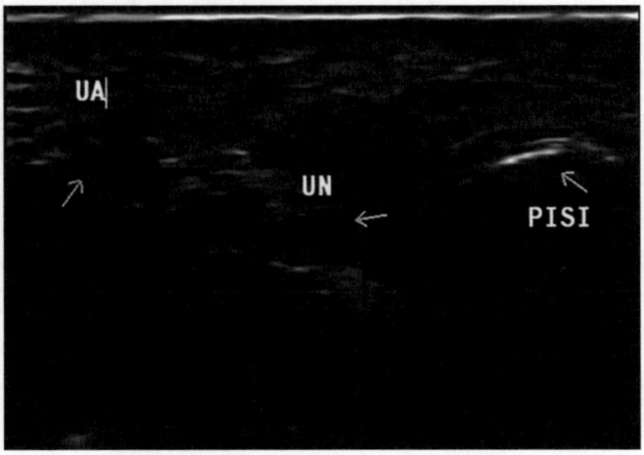

Figure 8.
Short-axis scan of the ulnar nerve (UN) at Guyon's canal. PISI. Pisiform bone; UA, ulnar artery.

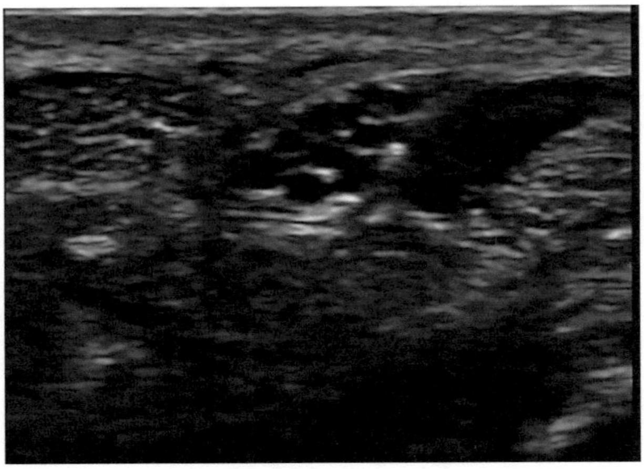

Figure 9.
Short-axis scan of the median nerve at the carpal tunnel.

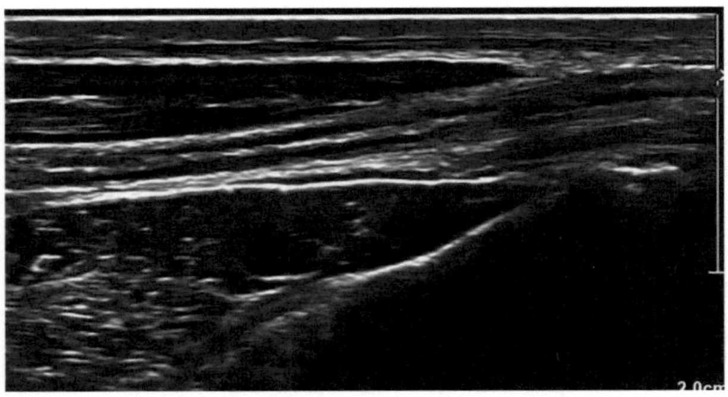

Figure 10.
Long-axis scan of the median nerve at the carpal tunnel.

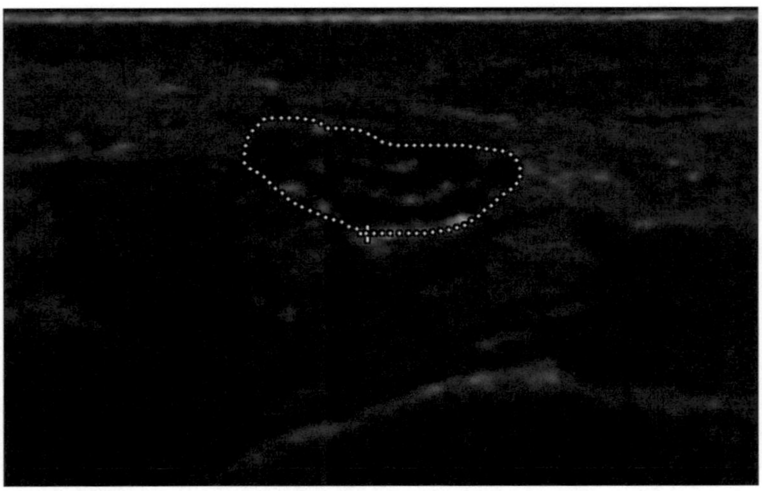

Figure 11.
Short-axis scan of the median nerve at the carpal tunnel with increased CSA.

one of the common compressive neuropathies) and at Guyon's canal at the level of wrist joint (**Figure 8**). The median nerve is the most important nerve of the upper limb. It arises from the C6-T1 nerve roots. The median nerve is also the easiest nerve

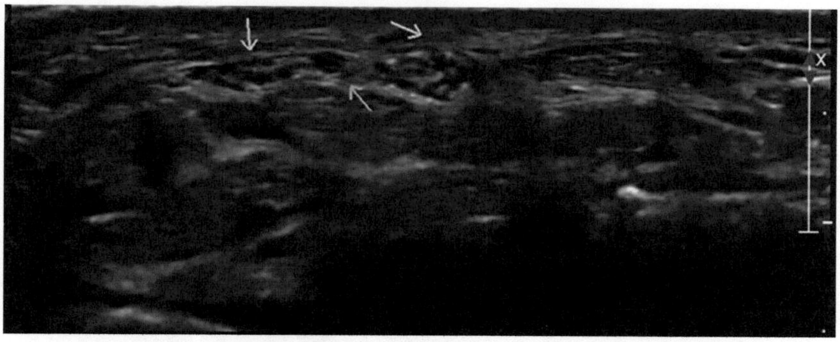

Figure 12.
Bifid median nerve at the level of the carpal tunnel.

scanned in the body. The commonest entrapment syndrome is related to this nerve when it entraps in the carpal tunnel level, the so called "carpal tunnel syndrome." Good knowledge about congenital anatomical variation is essential (**Figures 9–12**) [14, 15].

7. Lower limb nerves

The sensorimotor supply of the lower limb is derived from the lumbosacral plexus. The most important nerves of the lower limb are the sciatic nerve, the femoral nerve, the common fibular nerve, and the tibial nerve. Two other nerves could be added but are less important which are the saphenous nerve and the sural nerve. The femoral nerve could be injured during surgical/interventional procedures, and it gives branch to the saphenous nerve which also could be injured during varicose vein stripping operations due its close proximity to the long saphenous vein. The sciatic nerve is the largest nerve in the human. This nerve is practically a combination of the two nerves, the tibial and the fibular nerve with one common sheath. Actually the level of true division of the sciatic nerve into these nerves is highly variable in the human population (**Figures 13–15**) [14, 16].

8. Traumatic peripheral nerve injuries

Trauma to the peripheral nerves could be direct or indirect; one of the following consequences could happen. Structural and morphological changes could occur, resulting in change in the echogenicity or the shape of the nerve. Most of the studies take Sunderland classification as a reference to in dealing with the degree of

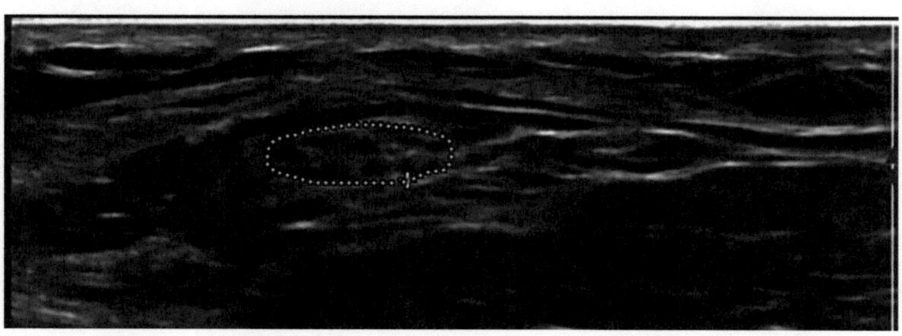

Figure 13.
Short-axis scan of the common fibular nerve.

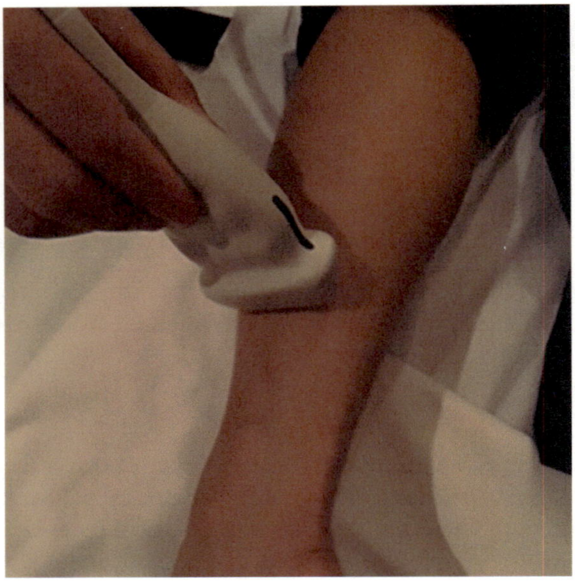

Figure 14.
Photo of scan of the sural nerve at the lateral aspect of leg.

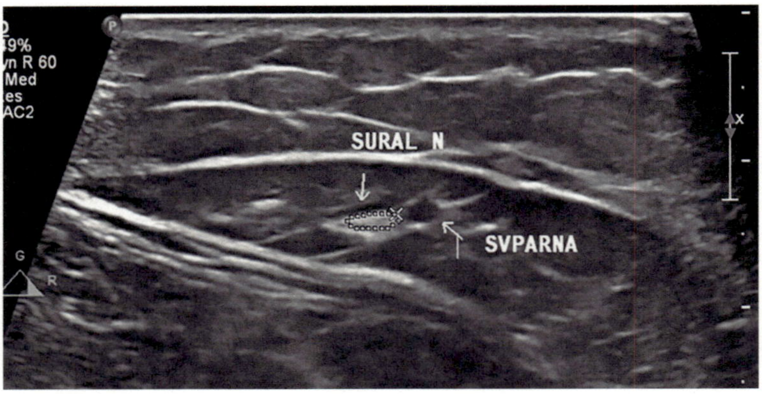

Figure 15.
Short-axis scan of the sural nerve at the lateral aspect of the leg.

post-traumatic peripheral nerve lesions. Penetrating injuries could lead to partial or complete cut of the nerve (transection), with associated laceration. One of the most important changes is nerve contusion and/or compression. Repetitive insults could lead to stretch along the course of the nerve. Ultrasound does not clearly demonstrate endoneurium but clearly visualize perineurium and epineurium. Also ultrasound could well demonstrate fascicular anatomy but not myelin and axonal anatomy [17]. In conclusion, the main role of ultrasound in the assessment of traumatic nerve lesions is to assess the continuity of the nerve and presence of axonotmesis or neurotmesis and also assessment of other sites of injury and, in some cases, the cause of injury.

Abbreviations

NCT	nerve conduction test
EMG	electromyography

MRI	magnetic resonance imaging
DTI	diffuse tensor imaging
CSA	cross-sectional area

Author details

Mohamed A. Bedewi[1]*, Daniele Coraci[2] and Sherine Swify[3]

1 Department of Internal Medicine, Prince Sattam Bin Abdulaziz University, College of Medicine, Alkharj, Kingdom of Saudi Arabia

2 Fondazione Policlinico A. Gemelli IRCCS, Rome, Italy

3 Ministry of Health and Population, Alexandria, Egypt

*Address all correspondence to: mohamedbedewi@yahoo.com

References

[1] Walker FO, Cartwright MS, Alter KE, Visser LH, Hobson-Webb LD, Padua L, et al. Indications for neuromuscular ultrasound: Expert opinion and review of the literature. Clinical Neurophysiology. December 2018;**129**(12):2658-2679

[2] Bedewi MA, Nissman D, Aldossary NM, Maetani TH, El Sharkawy MS, Koura H. Shear wave elastography of the brachial plexus roots at the interscalene groove. Neurological Research. September 2018;**40**(9):805-810

[3] Rangavajla G, Mokarram N, Masoodzadehgan N, Pai SB, Bellamkonda RV. Noninvasive imaging of peripheral nerves. Cells, Tissues, Organs. 2014;**200**(1):69-77

[4] Tagliafico A, Bignotti B, Tagliafico G, Martinoli C. Peripheral nerve MRI: Precision and reproducibility of T2*-derived measurements at 3.0-T: A feasibility study. Skeletal Radiology. May 2015;**44**(5):679-686

[5] Aggarwal A, Jana M, Srivastava DN, Sharma R, Gamanagatti S, Kumar A, et al. Magnetic resonance neurography and ultrasonogram findings in upper limb peripheral neuropathies. Neurology India. January-February 2019;**67**(Supplement):S125-S134

[6] Tagliafico AS. Peripheral nerve imaging: Not only cross-sectional area. World Journal of Radiology. August 2016;**8**(8):726-728

[7] Visalli C, Cavallaro M, Concerto A, La Torre D, Di Salvo R, Mazziotti S, et al. Ultrasonography of traumatic injuries to limb peripheral nerves: Technical aspects and spectrum of features. Japanese Journal of Radiology. October 2018;**36**(10):592-602. [Epub 2018 Aug 13, Review]

[8] Padua L, Di Pasquale A, Liotta G, Granata G, Pazzaglia C, Erra C, et al. Ultrasound as a useful tool in the diagnosis and management of traumatic nerve lesions. Clinical Neurophysiology. June 2013;**124**(6):1237-1243

[9] Zeidenberg J, Burks SS, Jose J, Subhawong TK, Levi AD. The utility of ultrasound in the assessment of traumatic peripheral nerve lesions: Report of 4 cases. Neurosurgical Focus. September 2015;**39**(3):E3

[10] Cartwright MS, Chloros GD, Walker FO, Wiesler ER, Campbell WW. Diagnostic ultrasound for nerve transection. Muscle & Nerve. June 2007;**35**(6):796-799

[11] Renna R, Coraci D, De Franco P, Erra C, Ceruso M, Padua L. Ultrasound study is useful to discriminate between axonotmesis and neurotmesis also in very small nerves: A case of sensory digital ulnar branch study. Medical Ultrasonography. December 2012;**14**(4):352-354 (Erratum in: Med Ultrason. 2013 Mar;15(1):78. Rosaria, Renna [corrected to Renna, Rosaria]; Daniele, Coraci [corrected to Coraci, Daniele])

[12] Bianchi ML, Padua L, Granata G, Erra C. Double site nerve lesion: Ultrasound diagnosed musculocutaneous involvement in traumatic brachial plexus injury. Clinical Neurophysiology. March 2013;**124**(3):629-630

[13] Zheng M, Zhu Y, Zhou X, Chen S, Cong R, Chen D. Diagnosis of closed injury and neoplasm of the brachial plexus by ultrasonography. Journal of Clinical Ultrasound. September 2014;**42**(7):417-422

[14] Kerasnoudis A, Pitarokoili K, Behrendt V, et al. Cross sectional area reference values for sonography

of peripheral nerves and brachial plexus. Clinical Neurophysiology. 2013;**124**:1881-1888

[15] Bedewi MA, Abodonya A, Kotb M, Mahmoud G, Kamal S, Alqabbani A, et al. Estimation of ultrasound reference values for the upper limb peripheral nerves in adults: A cross-sectional study. Medicine (Baltimore). December 2017;**96**(50):e9306

[16] Bedewi MA, Abodonya A, Kotb M, Kamal S, Mahmoud G, Aldossari K, et al. Estimation of ultrasound reference values for the lower limb peripheral nerves in adults: A cross-sectional study. Medicine (Baltimore). March 2018;**97**(12):e017

[17] Lauretti L, D'Alessandris QG, Granata G, Padua L, Roselli R, Di Bonaventura R, Fernandez E. Ultrasound evaluation in traumatic peripheral nerve lesions: From diagnosis to surgical planning and follow-up Acta Neurochirurgica (Wien). November 2015;**157**(11):1947-1951. discussion 1951

Chapter 4

Orthotic Treatment Overview of Carpal Tunnel Syndrome

Hasan Md Arif Raihan, Poly Ghosh, Prasanna Lenka, Ameed Equbal and Abhishek Biswas

Abstract

Carpal tunnel syndrome or median compressive neuropathy at the wrist is the condition of median nerve compression. Most of the CTSs are idiopathic and are provoked by repetitive grasping and manipulating activities, and the exposure can be cumulative. Orthotic splinting is prescribed both pre- and postsurgical but essentially in pre-surgical situation. The importance of wrist orthotic splints in non-operative treatment for carpal tunnel syndrome is a known scenario. Also evidentially it has a standard of care despite having varying rates of success. The aim and objective of orthotic splinting is to immobilize the wrist to stop flexion and maintain low range of wrist motion which help to decrease inflammation. CTS splint may be applied to dorsal side or in volar for maintaining wrist in a neutral position. The general recommendation is to wear a wrist immobilization orthotic splint as night splint. Splint kinematics and kinetics for biomechanical analyzing principles are essential to understand the principles involved in the various standard design, construction, and fitting of CTS splint. Application of orthotic biomechanics is for possessing a specific understanding of orthotic splinting function as per clinical orthotic assessment.

Keywords: carpal tunnel syndrome, orthotic splints, CTS biomechanics, CTS orthotic splint biomechanics

1. Introduction

Compression of the median nerve at the wrist is the most common upper extremity compressive neuropathy known as carpal tunnel syndrome [1–4]. It affects as much as 3% of the population at any one time. Still CTS remains a clinical syndrome, and as many as 15% of patients in some series have clinical evidence. Although surgical relieved for the median nerve compression my processed in the presence of normal severe electro diagnostic results [2, 3].

CTS decreases the cross-sectional area of the carpal tunnel that produces increased carpal tunnel canal volume content which may result in increased pressure in the carpal canal. Secondarily intracarpal tunnel pressure may be affected by external pressure to the palm [3].

The value of nonsurgical treatment protocol for mild CTS is a standard option. Conservative management is generally not an ideal option for moderate-to-severe CTS, especially in patients who have signs of muscle atrophy or significant sensory impairment. Non-surgery management options that have been described for CTS include orthosis use, nonsteroidal anti-inflammatory drugs, injection of the carpal tunnel with a corticosteroid, tendon-nerve gliding exercises, iontophoresis, ultrasound, and daily activity site modifications. The importance of CTS orthotic splints is well known in non-operative scenario. The American Academy of Neurology recommends a noninvasive orthotic treatment for the light and moderate CTS pathology. CTS orthotic treatment protocol remains the standard of care even though varying rates of success have been reported in the literature [5–7].

The objective of CTS splinting is immobilizing the wrist motion that decreases inflammation. Increased pressure in the carpal tunnel has been demonstrated with either wrist flexion or extension; therefore splinting of the wrist in a neutral position is recommended. Mild CTS symptoms of short duration are recommended with night splinting. Day and night splinting is recommended when there is mild-to-moderate symptoms during the day or with minimal activity. Also postoperative CTS splinting protects healing structures while allowing the predefined wrist motion.

Other significant objective of CTS splinting is ranging from pain relief and protection to prevention and correction of the wrist deformity.

Clinical orthotic assessment in terms of anatomic, kinesiology, neurology, and functional effects is important for prescribing CTS splint.

CTS and CTS splint's kinetics and kinematics analyses play a key role to understand the principles involved in the various standard design, construction, and fitting of CTS splint.

2. Orthotic assessment for CTS

Orthotic assessment includes the use of a variety of clinical qualitative and quantitative evaluation methods and instruments whose subsequent data is integrated to produce a clearly defined picture of CTS and its patho-biomechanics.

Points are essential for orthotic prescription.

- Demographic data and individual client factors (age, motivation, intelligence, vocation/avocation, clinic proximity).
- Chief complaint (type of pain during hand and wrist activity in static or dynamic condition).
- Previous orthotic treatment history (type of orthotic splint, function, and pressure system).
- Other treatment plans (postoperative, what are other medical conditions).
- Manual muscle testing (minimum gravity control muscle power for wrist patho-kinetics).
- Active range of motion (check the wrist patho-kinematics).
- Passive range of motion (check the wrist patho-kinematics).
- Upper extremity reflexes (check wrist pathophysiology).
- Skin condition (orthotic splint material).
- Body temperature (orthotic splint material and design).
- Perspiration (providing hole over orthotic splint).

- Soft tissue condition (check pressure tolerance capacity. Creep, stress-relaxation, stress rate sensitivity, etc.).
- Pain scale (VAS scale, which type of pain and how to grade pain according to splint pressure system applied).
- Clinical test related to CTS (diagnosis of abnormal motion and pain).
- X-ray finding (structure of carpal tunnel and any other involvement).
- Swelling (orthotic splint material for low-grade swelling).
- EMG test (muscle activity profile, resting potential, neuromuscular junction condition, neuromuscular integration for wrist joint kinetic and kinematic condonation).
- NCV-test (median nerve activity profile, resting potential, neuromuscular junction condition, neuromuscular integration for wrist joint kinetic and kinematic condonation).
- Coordination (central nervous to peripheral nerve activity through wrist joint kinematics for various activity of daily living).
- Dexterity (power and precision grip strength).
- Asking price (appropriate to individual client factors and third-party payers).
- Period of time splint is to be used (temporary, semipermanent, permanent).
- Minimalism (no irrelevant parts, splint is applicable and pertinent to the need).
- Optimum function (splint allows usage and performance without unnecessary reduction of motion).
- Optimal sensation (splint permits as much sensory input as possible).
- Efficient fabrication (no extraneous parts or procedures, such as the use of reinforcement parts instead of curving contour, bonding instead of uninterrupted coalescing of components, straps instead of contiguous fit, inappropriate use of padding).
- Application and removal (appropriate to individual client factors).
- Client suggestions (requested adaptations that would not alter or jeopardize splint function).
- Influencing primary and secondary joints (motion allowed or restricted appropriately; components accomplish intended functions).
- Attaining purpose (immobilize, mobilize, restrict motion, or transmit torque).
- Effect on joints not included in splint; kinetic effects (avoids application of contraindicated forces to no splinted joints).

- Anatomical variables (surface of application appropriate, healing structures protected as necessary, external hardware considered).
- Exercise routine (permits efficient execution of prescribed therapeutic exercises).
- Patient education.

Orthotic assessment is essential for the splinting design program and instructions for the wearing times and exercise regimen, donning and doffing, and precautions.

3. CTS-ASHT orthotic splint nomenclature

American Society of Hand Therapists, ASHT (SCS) (1989), developed a universal splint nomenclature. It is based on splint function rather than splint design.

CTS splint classification also follows this classification. SCS components consist of identification of articular/nonarticular, location, direction, purpose (immobilization, mobilization, restriction, torque transmission), type, and the total number of joints. All splints have inherent mechanical characteristics that combine to a series of predictable patterns [1–3].

3.1 Articular/nonarticular orthotic splint

The principal division is given below (**Tables 1–6**).

Articular splints for CTS follow three-point/four-point or two-point pressure systems to affect the wrist joint by immobilizing, mobilizing, restricting, or transmitting torque. Nonarticular splints for CTS mainly obey the two-point pressure forces to stabilize or immobilize the wrist joint.

ESCS splint classification system (ESCS) for CTS splint groupings of primary and secondary joints, when a primary joint is linked with its potential secondary joint partners, a predictable linear pattern (**Table 2**).

3.1.1 Examples

Joints = [elbow level] = type 1

Total joints = [wrist + elbow = 2 joints] = (2)

Articular/nonarticular orthotic splint	
Articular	Those that affect articular structures
Nonarticular	Those that affect an anatomic segment or structure but do not affect joint motion or cross a joint

Table 1.
Principal classification of orthotic splint.

Primary joints	Secondary joints			Total joint involvement/splint
Wrist joint	DIP	PIP	MP	Design and tramline of CTS splint (0 type, 1 type, 2 type, etc.)

Table 2.
CTS orthotic splint classification.

Force (KP)	Wrist flexion (degree)	Wrist extension (degree)
0–10	0–5	0–5
10–20	5–10	5–10
20–30	10–15	10–15
30–40	15–20	15–20

In force (KP) the resultant tendon force was 0–10, 10–20, 20–30, and 30–40. Wrist flexion (degree) had 0–5, 5–10, 10–15, and 15–20. Wrist extension (degree) had 0–50, 5–10, 10–15, and 15–20.

Table 3.
Resultant tendon force on wrist sagittal plane motion.

Study	Patients with CTS		
	Neutral position (mmHg)	Flexion (mmHg)	Extension (mmHg)
Gelberman et al. (1981)	32 ± 4.27	94 ± 12.53	110 ± 14.66
Werener et al. (1983)	31 ± 4.13	75 ± 10	105 ± 14
Szabo and Chidgey (1989)	10 ± 1.33	32 ± 4.27	51 ± 6.80
Okutsu et al. (1989)	43 ± 5.73	192 ± 25.60	222 ± 29.60
Luchetti et al. (1989)	26 ± 3.47	—	—
Rojviroj et al. (1990)	12 ± 1.60	27 ± 3.60	33 ± 4.40
Graham et al. (1991)	20 ± 2.67	—	—

Table 4.
Reviewed report for wrist pressure in normal position, flexion position, and extension position.

Wrist position (sagittal and frontal planes) with minimum pressure (mmHg) in CTS splint		
	Minimum pressure	Wrist motion
CTS	19 ± 1.5	Flexion 2 ± 0.7 ulnar deviation 1 ± 0.4
Normal/CTS splint	8 ± 0.75	Extension 2 ± 0.7 ulnar deviation 2 ± 1

Table 5.
Minimum wrist pressure for CTS and wrist motion.

Carpal tunnel pressure (mmHg) data for subjects performing a repetitive material handling Task with and without a wrist splint							
Pre activity baseline		During activity		Post activity baseline		During activity	
Without splint	With splint	Without splint	With splint	Without splint	With splint	First minute of activity	Last minute of activity
6	5	13	12	6	5	12	13

Table 6.
Pressure of flexible wrist splint on carpal tunnel during repetitive hand activity.

4. Orthotic treatments for CTS

Orthotic splinting for CTS still remains the standard option [8–10]. CTS splint is mainly prescribed before surgery including muscle atrophy or continuous sensory impairment. Patients who present with mild symptoms will have the best option to conservative splinting.

Hence orthotic CTS splint is prescribed for mild-to-moderate and postoperative conditions.

Numerous customized design orthotic splints are commercially available. On the other hand, custom-fit CTS orthosis may be made for individual patients for minimizing external pressure over the median nerve.

Customized volar or dorsal orthotic splints are provided with neutral position over wrist joint. Dorsal-based splint Carpal Lock CTS splint applied for restricting kinematic external pressure over the carpal tunnel with thin straps over the palm leave the palmar surface free. It is indicated for mild CTS patient.

The general principle for orthotic splint application which maintains the wrist in a neutral position is that pressure on the median nerve as it passes through the carpal tunnel is amplified in positions of wrist flexion and extension (Gelberman 1984). Neutral wrist joint position (loose pack position) is the clinical condition for orthotic splinting to hold the wrist even when the patient is asleep and likely to flex their wrist without being able to correct themselves. The wrist angle in CTS splint and altering the shape of the carpal tunnel are moving the lumbricals distally out of the carpal tunnel to decrease pressure on the median nerve (Manente et al. 2001).

Manente et al. (2001) expressed a compared report for night CTS splint (4 weeks) with no treatment group. Premoselli et al. (2006) performed a quasi-randomized trial that compared a CTS splint worn at night for 6 months with no treatment group. Both studies concluded that orthotic splinting has a significant impact on CTS.

4.1 Static CTS wrist hand orthosis

WHO is the standard design option used in CTS. Wrist joint is one of the key elements for upper extremity splinting. Fine tune position of wrist splint maintains powerful extrinsic tendon, finger, and hand digital posture and motion. Static is indicated to make the wrist static and restrict sagittal and coronal plane motions.

Many plastics and metallic standard CTS-WHO splint are designed for orthotic treatment by various universities and institutes as the Institute in Chicago, the Institute for Rehabilitation and Research in Houston, and the Institute of Rehabilitation Medicine at New York University.

4.2 CTS immobilization splints

Wrist immobilization orthotic splint for CTS aimed to allow healing of injured or inflamed wrist. This splint can restrict sagittal and coronal plane motions. The correct application can provide significant result in mild-to-moderate CTS. For increasing mechanical advantage, two-thirds the length of the forearm extension may be added in CTS splint.

4.2.1 CTS immobilization splint type 0

- Here the primary joint of a type 0 wrist immobilization splint is the wrist itself.

- There are no secondary joints included in a type 0 wrist splint. Neutral wrist position is also used frequently, and, in this instance, the splint is called a wrist neutral immobilization splint, type 0.

4.2.2 CTS immobilization splint type 1

- Type 1 wrist immobilization splint indicates the presence of one secondary joint level included in the splint in addition to the primary joint, the wrist.
- The secondary joint most often included in a wrist immobilization splint, type 1 (2), is the thumb CMC joint, which is held motionless by a carefully fitted first metacarpal bar component.
- Type 1 wrist immobilization splints that include the thumb CMC may be used to help control and/or decrease wrist pain.
- Because mechanical purchase on the first metacarpal is challenging, complete immobilization of the CMC joint is difficult to achieve with a type 1 wrist immobilization splint.

4.2.3 CTS immobilization splint type 2

- Type 2 wrist immobilization splints incorporate two secondary joint levels in addition to the wrist the primary joint. Secondary joint(s) may be situated either proximal or distal to the wrist depending on the specific purpose of the splint.
- For example, splints may include both the thumb CMC and MP as distally located secondary joint levels, or they may include the forearm and elbow as proximal secondary level joints.
- Type 2 wrist immobilization splints that incorporate the thumb are sometimes used to provide additional stabilization for partial fusions or fractures on the radial side of the wrist including scaphoid fractures or radial wrist ligament injuries where thumb IP joint motion is permitted.

4.3 CTS mobilization splints

Generally prescribe for the postoperative CTS patients.

- Supple wrists that lack active motion.
- Stiff wrists with the limited passive range of motion. For the most part, flaccid wrists lacking full or partial active motion require simple mobilization splints that facilitate and improve hand function. Occasionally, more complicated splinting utilizing torque transmission may be required to substitute for absent movement in supple wrists. Types of CTS splints are type 0, type 1, and type 3.

4.4 CTS restriction splints

Restriction CTS orthotic splints are prescribed to acute mild CTS patients for daytime use for restricting or where defined arcs of active wrist motion are required. Prescribe for the pre- and postoperative CTS patients.

Wrist sagittal and coronal plane motion restriction is controlled by inflexible materials like thermoplastic, metal, etc. Less rigid materials like neoprene, leather, vinyl, and tape are used for some allowing some degree of wrist range of motion. CTS restriction splints are type 0 and type 2.

4.4.1 CTS restriction splints type 0

- Type 0 wrist restriction splints control motion at one primary joint the wrist. There are no secondary joints included in type 0 restriction splints.

- Restriction splints may be designed and fit to allow full or limited wrist extension/flexion while preventing radial and ulnar deviation or vice versa, or they may simply limit motion in one direction while allowing increments of motion in other directions.

- Wrist circumduction restriction splints allow varying degrees of overall wrist mobility while providing external support for sports, work, and/or avocational activities.

- These splints are constructed in softer materials including tape neoprene or fabric.

4.4.2 CTS restriction splints type 2

- Type 2 wrist restriction splints limit gradations of wrist motion and are used with a variety of diagnoses. They are often worn during sports or work activities.

- Generally, these splints allow normal motion while limiting extreme motion in extension and/or flexion or in radial and/or ulnar deviation.

- One of the most commonly used type 2 wrist restriction splints includes the thumb CMC and MP as secondary joints.

4.5 CTS torque transmission splints

These are usually prescribed in postoperative CTS patients. Dynamic splinting is not recommended for CTS patients. Postoperative CTS patients may be prescribed who are having patho-kinematics in the transverse plane (wrist rotation). Also it is used for the therapeutic approach for contracture release for CTS.

4.5.1 CTS torque transmission splints type 3 and type 4

- Torque transmission splints affecting the wrist joint may have three or four secondary joint levels incorporated and are categorized as type 3 or type 4, respectively.

- These splints function longitudinally by controlling finger joint motion to transmit torque to the wrist joint proximally so that extrinsic muscle power is focused exclusively on the wrist joint.

4.5.2 CTS dynamic splinting application

Berner et al. (2008) studied with dynamic splint application for a modality that treats CTS using low-load, prolonged duration stretch to reduce contracture, which contributes to median nerve compression. Dynamic splinting reduced experimental patients' symptoms and improved electrodiagnostic parameters [11] (**Figures 1–7**).

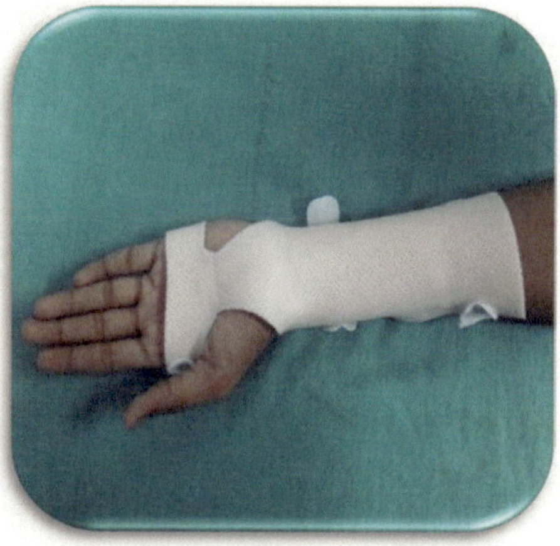

Figure 1.
CTS volar splint.

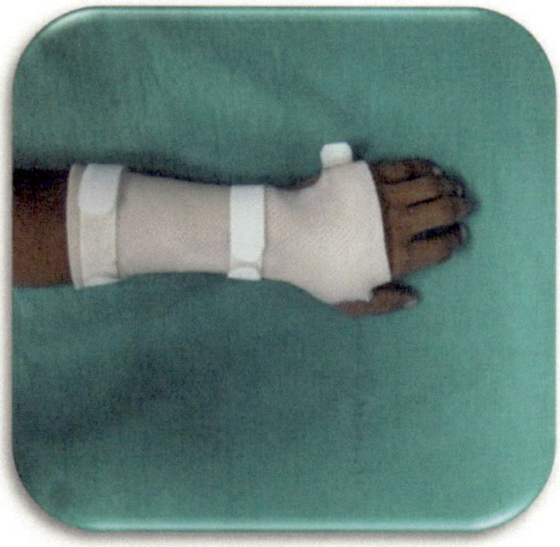

Figure 2.
CTS dorsal splint.

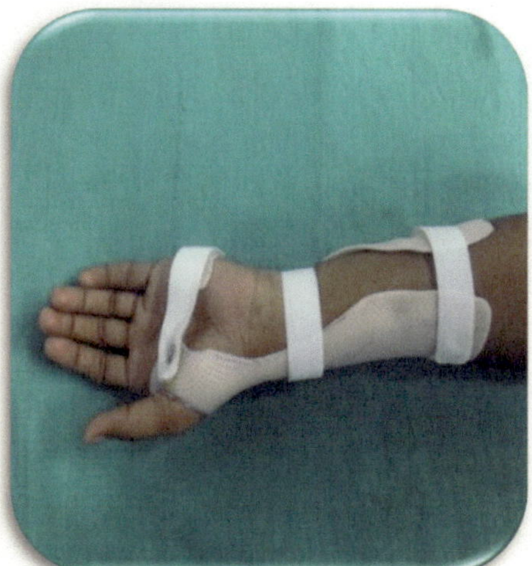

Figure 3.
CTS wrist hand orthosis with thumb extension.

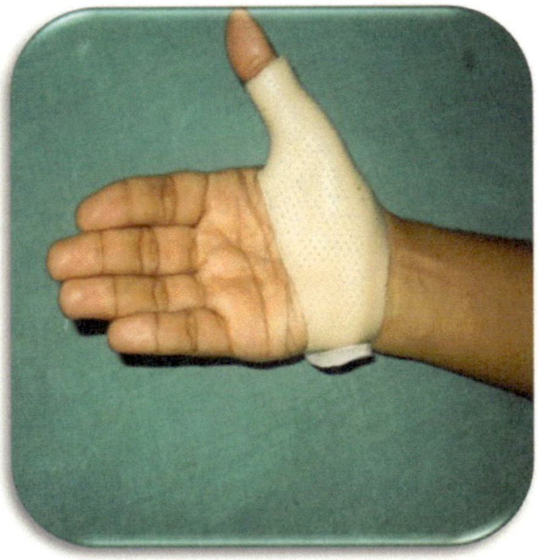

Figure 4.
CTS carpal lock splint.

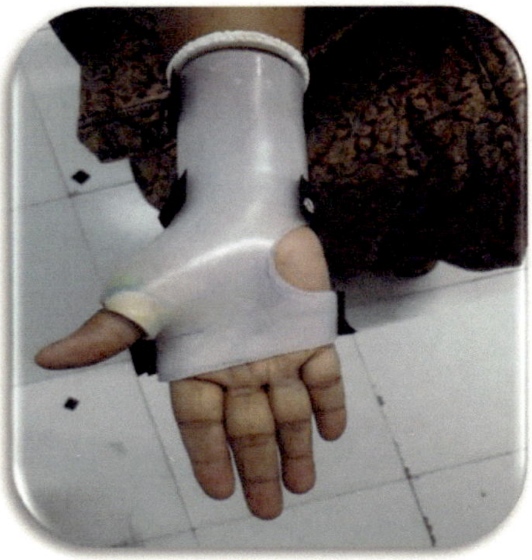

Figure 5.
CTS thumb spica.

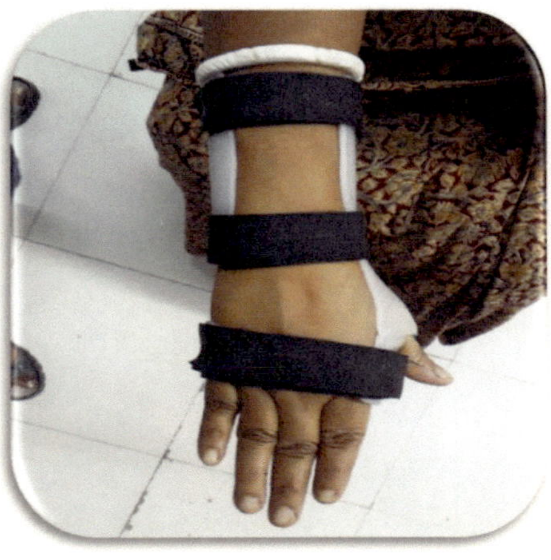

Figure 6.
CTS thumb spica.

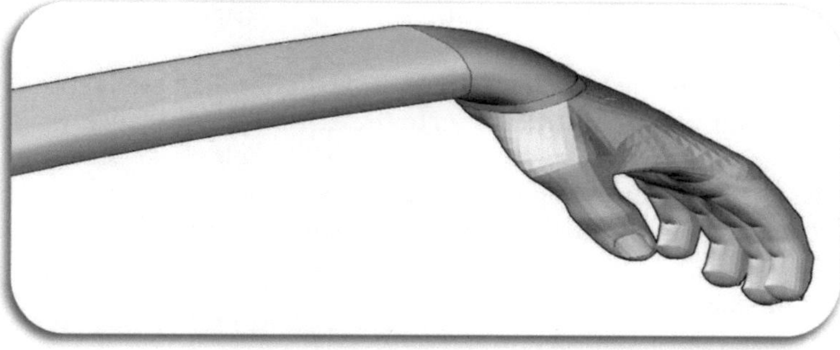

Figure 7.
Three-dimensional model of CTS hand.

5. Orthotic clinical checkout guidelines for CTS orthotic splinting

Given the diagnostic requirements the splint has been fitted appropriately to adapt to the following:

- Anatomical structure (bony prominences, arches, dual obliquity, skin creases).
- Ligamentous stress (immobilization, mobilization, restriction, or torque transmission forces correctly applied to avoid damage or attenuation).
- Joint alignment (anatomical axes aligned with splint articulation; splint does not shift inappropriately on extremity).
- Kinematic changes (splint does not inappropriately inhibit motion of unrestricted or partially restricted joints; splint does not inappropriately transmit torque).
- Contiguous fit of components on extremity.
- Good overall esthetic appearance.
- Corners rounded, edges and surfaces smooth and flanged appropriately.
- Joined surfaces stable and finished (bonds solid, securing devices of sufficient number and correctly applied; internal edges smoothed, securing devices finished).
- Ventilation (appropriately placed, splint strength not jeopardized).

6. Classical mechanical theories for CTS splint

Most splints used in upper extremity clinical practice apply consistent, linear-oriented, three-point pressure systems to affect joint motion. These splints incorporate three parallel reciprocal forces with the proximal and distal forces oriented in the same direction and the middle reciprocal force oriented in the opposite [6, 7, 12].

The diagnostic requirements, does the splint meet mechanical criteria, including adaptation.

6.1 Increase the area of force application

Pressure = total force/area of force application. Splinting materials are, to varying degrees, rigid; their improper application to the extremity may cause damage to the cutaneous surface and underlying soft tissue as a result of excessive pressure. Splint applies over bony prominences or in areas where the inherent structure of the splint influences to increase the pressure of mechanical counterforces.

6.2 Increase mechanical advantage

Splinting is acting like the lever system. Splint provides more mechanical advantage by the use of favorable force systems. The design and construction of splints significantly provide the mechanical advantages.

6.3 Use optimum rotational force

Splint restricts the compressive or tensile force through the mobilization (90° angle of approach to segments mobilized, perpendicular to joint axes) splint in stiffened joints through traction. Splint must be achieved without generating patient frustration or increased tissue damage. Two dimensions and three dimensions of force resolution are used for minimizing force load by the splint.

6.4 Consider the torque effect

Torque equals the product of the force times the length of the arm on which it acts. Patients may be taught to use the torque phenomenon advantageously by advancing their finger cuffs distally as their pain tolerance permits. The splint should be provided opposite torque for neutralization of torque effect.

6.5 Consider the relative degree of passive mobility of successive joints

Primary and secondary joints are responsible for maintaining static and dynamic equilibrium. When motion is limited or stopped at a given articulation, the remaining mobile joints are moved in the direction of the force with minimal motion occurring at the restricted.

6.6 Control reaction effect at secondary joints

The amount of stiffness between primary and secondary joints within the same longitudinal segment is marked; as a mobilization force is directed to a stiff joint and reciprocal force secondary joint motion is controlled, the end of the stabilized segment may have a tendency to displace or sublux at the level of the secondary joint.

6.7 Consider the effects of reciprocal parallel forces

The use of three parallel forces in equilibrium is achieved in the splint by two-point, three-point, or four-point pressure system.

6.8 Increase material strength by providing contour

Proper contour of splinting provides better controls of forces equilibrium in 3 dimensional plane.

6.9 Appropriate components

Parallel to providing elements of control and motion, articulated splints defend healing of soft tissue structures and improve function. Articulated splint mechanisms must be accurately aligned with anatomical joint axes. If a splint articulation is not aligned with its anatomical joint, the splint tends to the piston on the extremity as active movement occurs, causing shear forces and friction.

6.10 Eliminate friction

Kinetic friction develops when surfaces in contact with each other move relative to one another. If a difference in density exists between the surfaces, the harder surface may begin to erode the softer, less dense surface. If the surfaces are similar, damage may occur on either side or on both sides.

6.11 Avoid high shear stress

The important terms describe the material behavior of soft tissues.

7. Biomechanics of CTS

Quantitative biomechanical analysis of CTS is for finding how internal external forces/pressure inside flexed and extended wrists is related to wrist size hand force and hand position. Analyzing pathological condition of CTS is helpful for finding causes of wrist deformity and wrist pain. Biomechanics analysis is involved for finding deformed boney three-dimensional alignment, muscle devotion, deformed nerve condition, and ligament tendon pathological changes.

7.1 Biomechanical reflection for CTS

Biomechanics of CTS is playing an important role for proper application of CTS splinting. Here some kinematics and kinetic are discussed as per previous analysis.

Muscle force of extrinsic finger flexor muscles and flexor digitorum profundus and superficial and the flexor pollicis longus muscles that are providing effort force to the hand. Additionally forearm muscle forces are acting to the fingers with long tendons that pass through the carpal tunnel. Flexor retinaculum reinforced to wrist tendons in wrist flexion condition and in wrist extension condition tendons are reinforced by carpal bones.

Armstrong and Chaffin, 1978, found that the deviation of the wrist from the straight position causes the extrinsic finger flexor tendons to be displaced against, and past, the adjacent walls of the carpal tunnel.

7.2 Kinetic model of CTS wrist

Le Veau et al. 1974 also found that the tendon sliding over a curved surface is analogous to a belt draped around a pulley.

The force FL, exerted on a pulley, is a function of the belt tension Ft; the radius of the pulley curvature, r; the coefficient of friction between the pulley and the belt, μ; and the included angle of pulley-belt contact, α, and is expressed.

$$\text{FL Force (force/Arch length)} = \text{Fte}\ \mu\,\alpha/\text{r} \tag{1}$$

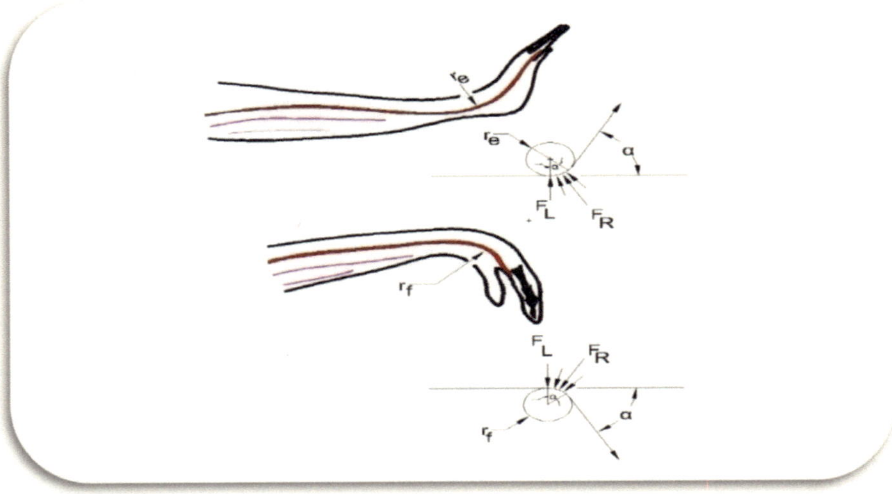

Figure 8.
2D force calculation for CTS.

Linn et al. (1968) and Linn and Radin et al. (1968) found that the coefficient of tendon-trochlear friction has not been measured directly; however, friction measurements of surfaces lubricated with bovine synovial fluid indicate that the coefficient would be in the range of 0.01–0.1.

For coefficients of friction in this range, friction can be neglected without greatly affecting force estimates; thus Eq. (1) can be approximated by

$$FL = Ft/r \quad (2)$$

Equation (2) indicates that the tendon load is approximately uniformly distributed over the trochlea.

- Tendon load per unit length as a function of tendon curvature and load.
- It can be seen that the contact force between the tendons and trochlea increases directly with tendon tension and inversely with the radius of tendon curvature.
- The radius of curvature can be estimated for different wrist thicknesses (Armstrong and Chaffin, 1978); the tendon tension can be estimated for given positions of given sized hands (Dempster, 1961; Smith et al., 1964; Chao et al., 1976; Armstrong, 1976) (**Figures** 7 and **8**).

It has been suggested that force between the extrinsic finger flexor tendons and the trochlea in the flexed wrist compresses the median nerve and is a factor of carpal tunnel syndrome (Brain et al., 1949; Robbins, 1963; Phalen, 1966).

- Compression of the median nerve by adjacent tendons has been confirmed by direct pressure measurements at the site of the median nerve by Tanzer (1959) and by Smith et al. (1977).
- In addition to the median nerve, the synovial membranes of the radial and ulnar bursas that surround the extrinsic finger flexor tendons are compressed by forces in both flexed and extended wrists. It has been suggested that repeated compression can lead to synovial inflammation and swelling,

which in turn leads to compression of the median nerve inside the carpal tunnel (Yamaguchi et al., 1965; Phalen, 1966, 1972; Tichauer, 1966, 1975, 1976).

- Armstrong et al. (1979) suggest that the resultant force is exerted by a tendon on adjacent wrist structures as a function of wrist angle and tendon load. The resultant force is independent of tendon and wrist size [13].

- Thomas J. et al. (1979) found that the CTS resultant force is exerted by a tendon on adjacent wrist structures as a function of wrist angle and tendon load. The resultant force is independent of tendon and wrist size (**Table 3**).

8. Kinematics and kinetics of orthotic CTS splint

Biomechanics of CTS splint is for analyzing the kinematics and kinetics of wrist with splinting. Kinematics analysis signifies the wrist range of motion, and kinetics analysis signifies wrist pressures with splinting. Many studies were performed on kinematics and kinetics of CTS splint. Here we summarized the previous results for finding range of motion and wrist pressure with splinting condition.

Keir et al. (1999) found the direction of determining MRI for tendon paths has provided new insight into the relationships between the finger flexor tendons and other structures at the wrist [14].

Weiss et al. (1995) reviewed the wrist pressure in the normal position, flexion position, and extension position [15] (**Table 4**).

- Weiss ND and Gordon et al. (1995) also found that the minimum wrist pressure for CTS is to be maintained in CTS splint with limited range of motion (**Table 5**).

- Di Domizio et al. (2008) found that when the splint was used, there was a significant reduction in extensor carpi radialis ECR and flexor carpi radialis FCR activity. That was presumably due to participants' use of the splint to support some of the load that would be expected in the radial muscles to counteract gravity given that the standard posture required a neutral forearm and no radioulnar deviation [16].

- Rempel et al. (1994) found the pressure of flexible wrist splint on carpal tunnel during repetitive hand activity [17] (**Table 6**).

Acknowledgements

Authors would like to thank Mr. Ananda Poddar, Project Assistance, Department of Rehabilitation Engineering; and also thank Mr. B.B.Bharti (MPO), Mr. SamirSamanta (MPO), Miss RashmitaDash (MPO), Miss Smurti Sahoo (MPO), Mr. HarshKumar (MPO), Miss Subhlata (MPO), Miss Shaliny (MPO), Mr. Subhasish (MPO), Mr. Mirtunjay (MPO), and Mr. Aryan (MPO), Department of Prosthetics and Orthotics, NILD, Kolkata.

Conflict of interest

No conflict of interest. Authors are donning clinical practice and clinical research for updated teaching.

Author details

Hasan Md Arif Raihan*, Poly Ghosh, Prasanna Lenka, Ameed Equbal and Abhishek Biswas
The West Bengal University of Health Sciences, National Institute for Locomotor Disabilities, Kolkata, India

*Address all correspondence to: arifraihan7@gmail.com

References

[1] Mansivias JJ, Bucher PA, Monsvias DB. Nonsurgically treated carpal tunnel syndrome in the manual worker. Plastic and Reconstructive Surgery. 1994;**94**:695-699

[2] Rempel D, Maojilovic R, Levinsohn DG, Bloom T, Gordon L. The effect of wearing a flexible wrist splint on carpal tunnel pressure during repetitive hand activities. The Journal of Hand Surgery. 1994;**19A**:106-110

[3] Sailer SM. The role of splinting and rehabilitation in the treatment of carpal and cubital tunnel syndromes. Hand Clinics. 1996;**12**:223-241

[4] Available from: http://www.360oandp.com/about-360-o-and-p.aspx

[5] Fess EE. Splint Mechanical Patterns©, Presented to the ASHT Splint Nomenclature Task Force, January, 1991. American Society of Hand Therapists Splint Classification System; 1991

[6] Fess EE, Gettle KS, Strickland JW. Hand Splinting: Principles and Methods. 1st ed. St. Louis: Mosby; 1981

[7] Fess EE, Philips CA. Hand Splinting: Principles and Methods. ed 2 ed. St. Louis: Mosby; 1987

[8] Brand PW. Repetitive Stress on Insensitive Feet. Carville, LA: United States Public Health Service Hospital; 1975

[9] Brand PW. Clinical Mechanics of the Hand. St. Louis: Mosby; 1985

[10] Brand PW, Hollister A. Clinical Mechanics of the Hand. 2nd ed. St. Louis: Mosby; 1993

[11] Berner SH, Willis FB, Martinez J. Treating carpal tunnel syndrome with dynamic splinting: A randomized controlled trial. PM&R. 2008;**1**(1):1

[12] Brand PW, Hollister A. Clinical Mechanics of the Hand. 3rd ed. St. Louis: Mosby; 1999

[13] Armstrong TJ, Chaffin DB. Some biomechanical aspects of the carpal tunnel. Journal of Biomechanics. 1979;**12**(7):567-570

[14] Keir PJ, Wells RP. Changes in geometry of the finger flexor tendons in the carpal tunnel with wrist posture and tendon load: An MRI study on normal wrists. Clinical Biomechanics. 1999;**14**(9):635-645

[15] Weiss ND, Gordon L, Bloom T, So Y, Rempel DM. Position of the wrist associated with the lowest carpal-tunnel pressure: implications for splint design. Journal of Bone and Joint Surgery. 1995;**77**(11):1695-1699

[16] Wade A. A Physiological and Performance Comparison between a Traditional and Novel Tennis Grip; 2015

[17] Rempel D, Manojlovic R, Levinsohn DG, Bloom T, Gordon L. The effect of wearing a flexible wrist splint on carpal tunnel pressure during repetitive hand activity. The Journal of Hand Surgery. 1994;**19**(1):1, 106-110

Chapter 5

Biological and Preclinical Evaluations of Designed Optically Guided Medical Devices with Light Scattering Modules for Carpal Tunnel Syndrome Treatment and Surgical Procedure

Ching-Cheng Huang and Ming-Che Chiang

Abstract

A novel technique and product applied to carpal tunnel microscopic surgical procedures through the designed medical devices were prepared and studied. The novel design of the medical device could be developed and applied for new carpal tunnel microscopic surgical procedures instead of the traditional carpal tunnel surgical procedures. Also, a new medical device with optical LLLT module was designed for wound healing in carpal tunnel syndrome treatments. Furthermore, assistive surgical healing dressings for carpal tunnel syndrome treatments via minimally invasive surgery (MIS) such as air-foam soft cleaning sponges and hydrogel surgical dressings with polymeric films were designed for more comfortable treatments. Biological and clinical evaluations of carpal tunnel surgical procedure using the new designed medical devices are studied. For commercialized reasons, guidance such as ISO 10993-1:2009(E) for biological evaluation of medical devices must be considered. Furthermore, the clinical evaluation of modified medical devices would be carried out.

Keywords: clinical evaluation, carpal tunnel syndrome, surgical procedure, minimally invasive surgery, scalpel

1. Introduction

Novel optically guided medical devices were designed for the clinical needs of carpal tunnel surgical procedure. The word "carpus" means "wrist." The wrist is the joint between your hand and the lower part of your arm and is surrounded by a band of fibrous tissue as a support for the joint. The tight space between the wrist bone and the fibrous band is called the carpal tunnel. The median nerve could pass through the carpal tunnel to receive any kind of sensations from the thumb, index, and middle fingers of the hand. Hence, any condition that causes swelling or a change in position of the tissue within the carpal tunnel would repress and damage the median nerve. Repression and irritation of the median nerve would cause numbness and tingling of the thumb, index, and the middle fingers of the hand which is a clinical condition known as "carpal tunnel syndrome." Although it is a gradual process, for most people carpal tunnel syndrome will worsen over time without some form of treatment. For this reason, it is important to be evaluated and diagnosed by doctor early on. In the early stages, it may be possible to slow or stop the progression of carpal tunnel syndrome. Two kinds of treatments could be employed in the stages such as nonsurgical treatments and surgical treatments. If diagnosed and treated early, the symptoms can often be relieved without surgery. If diagnosis is uncertain or if symptoms are mild, nonsurgical treatment would be recommend first. The nonsurgical treatments may include wearing a brace or splint at night; keeping the wrist in a straight or neutral position reduces pressure on the nerve in the carpal tunnel. It may also be useful to wear a splint during the day when doing activities that aggravate symptoms. In addition, nonsurgical treatments may include using the medical devices with light, electrode, etc. Also, nonsteroidal anti-inflammatory drugs (NSAIDs) could be a chosen way for nonsurgical treatments. Some medical devices such as photo- and electrotherapies could help relieve pain and inflammation for carpal tunnel syndrome. Furthermore, nerve gliding exercises, activity changes, and steroid injections would also be recommended as kinds of nonsurgical treatments for carpal tunnel syndrome. About nerve gliding exercises, some patients would benefit from exercises of nonsurgical treatments that help the median nerve move more freely within the confines of the carpal tunnel. About activity changes, symptoms often occur when the hand and wrist are in the same position for too long—particularly when the wrist is extended or flexed. About steroid injections, corticosteroid or cortisone is a powerful anti-inflammatory agent that could be injected into the carpal tunnel. If nonsurgical treatment could not relieve or stop the progression of carpal tunnel syndrome after a period of time, surgical treatments of carpal tunnel syndrome such as "carpal tunnel release" would be recommended and employed. Open carpal tunnel release could be employed as a kind of surgical treatment. In open surgery, a small incision must be made in the palm of target hand and views the inside of your hand and wrist through this incision [1]. During the procedure, the transverse carpal ligament will be divided in the roof of the carpal tunnel. This increases the size of the tunnel and decreases pressure on the median nerve. When the ligament heals after surgery, there is more room for the nerve and tendons. The other way, endoscopic carpal tunnel release was employed. In endoscopic surgery, one or two smaller skin incisions must be obtained and called portals for using an endoscope to observe inside target hand and wrist. A special knife is used to divide the transverse carpal ligament, similar to the open carpal tunnel release procedure [1].

In this report, we propose a series of novel techniques and medical devices of treatments for carpal tunnel syndrome. The novel design of the medical device could be developed and applied for new carpal tunnel microscopic surgical procedures instead of the traditional carpal tunnel surgical procedures. For the design of new medical devices, selections of materials or suitable materials for biomedical applications such as polymethacrylate, polyester, polyamide, polyimide, polyester, polynorbornene, polytetrafluoroethylene, polydiphenylacetylenes, and polymeric resins could be substantially considered and employed [1–19]. Also, the surface modification technology could be considered to change the surface microenvironment of materials for specific need [20–24]. Furthermore, the biological and clinical evaluations of materials and medical devices must be considered for the application and design.

2. Materials and methods

2.1 A new design of optical guided medical device with an electrical scalpel

New designed optical guided medical device with an electrical scalpel and a light scattering module was studied. The optical guided medical device with an electrical scalpel and a light scattering module contains a scalpel with a blade, an optical guided system with a scattering propagation, a power controller, and a connectable power supplier (**Figure 1**) [1].

2.2 A new design of laser optical guided medical device with a scalpel

New designed optical guided medical device with a scalpel was studied. Laser light sources could be employed as optical guided modules, and a series of laser optical guided medical devices with a scalpel are designed on the demands of clinical applications. The laser optical guided medical device with a scalpel contains a scalpel with a blade, an optical guided laser source with a designed strengthen arm, a power controller, and a connectable power supplier (King-Yard Tech. Co., TW). The different colors of laser light could be chosen depending on the clinical demands (**Figure 2**) [2, 3].

2.3 Assistive surgical healing dressings for carpal tunnel syndrome treatments via minimally invasive surgery(MIS): air-foam soft cleaning sponges and hydrogel surgical dressings with polymeric films

An air-foam soft cleaning sponge was designed for deeply soft cleaning the surgical skins before and after carpal tunnel syndrome treatments (Parsd Pharm. Tech. Co., TW) (**Figure 3**). The high medical grade Cenefom PVA raw sheet is a synthetic sponge essentially composed of cross-linked polyvinyl alcohol (PVA) through an air-foaming process, which could provide characteristics of lint-free and fiber-free, high hydrophilic, low chemical residues, and high cleanness of air-foam soft cleaning sponges. The sponges would be employed as assistive anti-adhesion dressings and satisfied for carpal tunnel syndrome treatments via minimally invasive surgery. The designed soft cleaning sponges must be a kind of open-celled microstructure, highly absorbent porous medical material that wicks aqueous solutions quickly. Their high-water content allows vapor and oxygen transmission to the wounds such as pressure sores, leg ulcers, surgical and necrotic wounds, lacerations, and burns. They seem to play an important role as emergency burns treatment alone or in combination with other products, thanks to their cooling and hydrating effects.

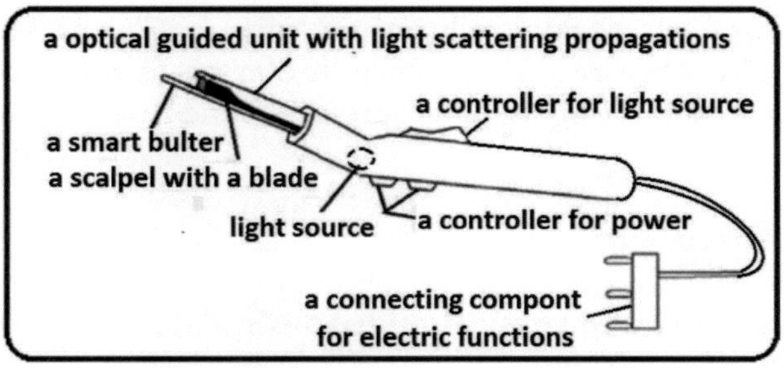

Figure 1.
New design of optical guided medical device with scalpel and its key functional components [1].

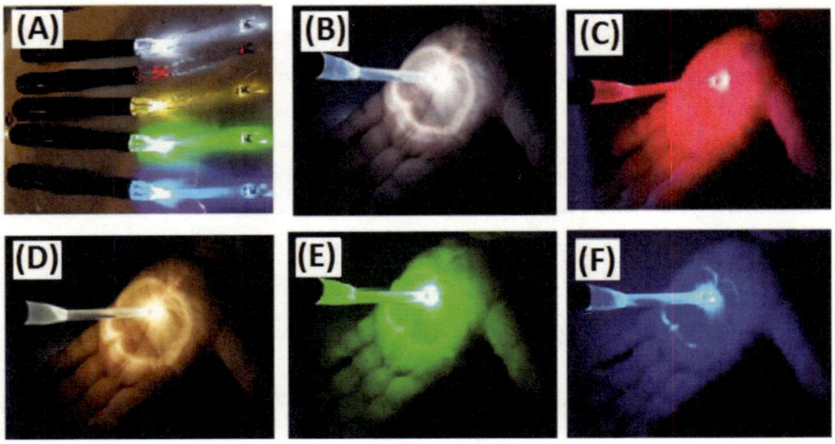

Figure 2.
(A) A series of new designed laser guided medical devices with a scalpel and different colors of laser light sources for various clinical demands (King-Yard Tech./Chuang Sheng Medicine Equipment Co., TW). (B) The white light focus on a hand, (C) the red light focus on a hand, (D) the orange light focus on a hand, (E) the green light focus on a hand, and (F) the blue light focus on a hand.

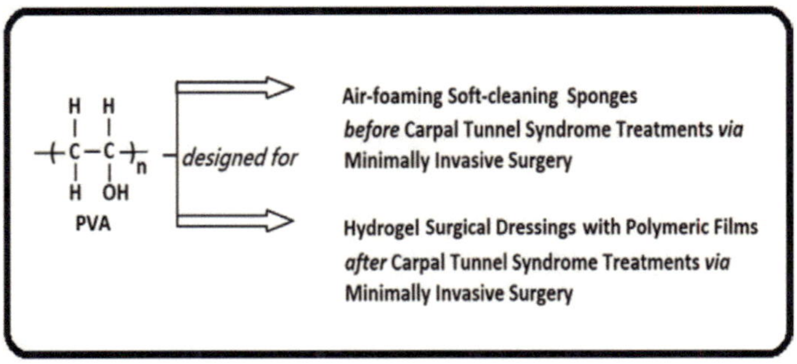

Figure 3.
Assistive surgical healing dressings for carpal tunnel syndrome treatments via minimally invasive surgery: air-foam soft cleaning sponges and hydrogel surgical dressings with polymeric films such as PU films.

In sual, the cross-linked or non-cross-linked polyvinyl alcohol (PVA) was employed to prepare hydrogel surgical dressings. The polyurethane film was used to be a protecting material, practically, for surgical dressings. The new surgical dressings were designed with well-protecting and surgical wound healing functions, which could provide good surgical wound managements after carpal tunnel syndrome treatments via minimally invasive surgery. That is, the hydrogel surgical dressing with a polymeric film was designed for the outside surgical wound healing after carpal tunnel syndrome treatments via minimally invasive surgery (Chuang Sheng Medicine Equipment Co., TW) (**Figure 3**). The polymeric film was used with the hydrogel surgical dressing for protecting the outer surgical wound from environments.

3. Results and discussion

3.1 New design of fabrication optical guided medical device with scalpel for carpal tunnel syndrome

In this study, traditional and conventional medical methods for carpal tunnel surgical procedure were modified, and novel optical guided medical device with scalpel was designed for carpal tunnel syndrome. For clinical demand, new design and fabrication of optical guided medical device with scalpel were necessary. Some essential components could be considered for the clinical need for carpal tunnel surgical procedure. Therefore, a new medical device was designed and had optically guided components with scalpel including a scalpel with a blade, an optically guided system with scattering propagation, a power controller, and a connectable power supplier (**Figure 1**). An individual head containing a surgical scalpel and an optically guided system could be considered in this study. Practically, the scattering propagation could be achieved by using the design of multiple stages in the optical guided cutting component [1]. Furthermore, the electrical supply, which could provide the function of optical guidance and electric cutting, was also considered as one part of the medical device as shown in **Figure 1**. The relative large operating area would be observed by traditional carpal tunnel surgical procedures as shown, respectively, in **Figure 4A**. Furthermore, the fabrication optical guided medical device with scalpel for carpal tunnel syndrome was carried out, and the new medical device could be used for carpal tunnel syndrome as shown in **Figure 4B–E**. The new designed light laser guided medical devices with a scalpel were employed in carpal tunnel surgical procedure (**Figure 4F**).

3.2 Characterization of the designed optical guided medical device with scalpel

The modified medical devices containing a head as a surgical scalpel under optical guidance were designed, and the newly designed head as a surgical scalpel was shown in **Figure 1**. The multiple stages for light scattering propagations were designed. The light scattering propagation occur because of the light transfer delay among different light waves, which satisfy the clinical demand during carpal tunnel surgical procedure to show the light pass route under the skin [1]. The polyacrylate was designed as a material for optical guidance instead of glass. The thermal deformation temperature was obtained as 93.9°C under 0.455 MPa (ASTM D648-07B). The new designed laser guided medical devices with a scalpel and a green light source was employed in carpal tunnel surgical procedure as shown in **Figure 4F**. The designed strengthen arm of medical devices increases the safety of carpal tunnel syndrome treatments via minimally invasive surgery. The surgery treatments would produce internal and external surgical damages. **Figure 5A** showed the surgical wounds of internal and external surgical damage after traditional carpal tunnel syndrome treatments. Comparably, **Figure 5B** showed the surgical wounds of internal and external surgical damage after the carpal tunnel syndrome

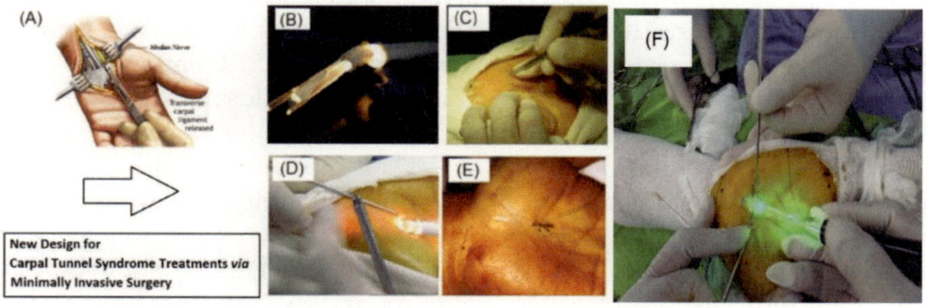

Figure 4.
Photos of (A) traditional design of medical devices for carpal tunnel surgical procedure (http://www.medicinenet.com/carpal_tunnel_syndrome/article.htm), (B) new design of optical guided medical device with scalpel in this study, and (C)–(E) new design of optical guided medical device with scalpel was employed in carpal tunnel surgical procedure. (F) The new designed light laser guided medical devices with a scalpel were employed in carpal tunnel surgical procedure.

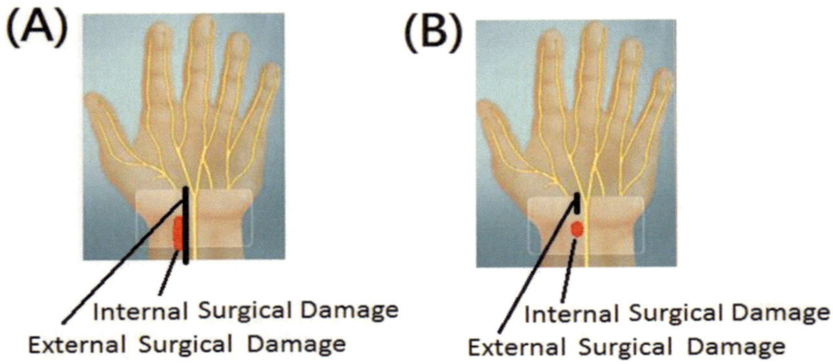

Figure 5.
(A) The surgical wounds of internal and external surgical damage after traditional carpal tunnel syndrome treatments and (B) the surgical wounds of internal and external surgical damage after the carpal tunnel syndrome treatments via minimally invasive surgery.

treatments via minimally invasive surgery with new designed laser guided medical devices. Remarkably, the relative small surgical wounds could be obtained by using new designed laser guided medical devices.

3.3 Characterization of the designed assistive dressings of air-foaming soft cleaning surgical sponge before carpal tunnel syndrome treatments via minimally invasive surgery

The surgical wounds of internal and external surgical damage would be observed after the carpal tunnel syndrome treatments whether the new designed laser guided medical devices via minimally invasive surgery or not (**Figure 5A** and **B**). For the specific clinical demands, designed assistive dressings of air-foaming soft cleaning surgical sponge must be designed before carpal tunnel syndrome treatments via minimally invasive surgery. The air-foaming soft cleaning PVA surgical sponge was prepared. The air-foaming soft cleaning PVA surgical sponge is a kind of synthetic sponge essentially composed of cross-linked polyvinyl alcohol, which was employed as assistive anti-adhesion dressings for carpal tunnel syndrome treatments via minimally invasive surgery. It is a kind of open-celled microstructure, highly absorbent porous material that wicks aqueous solutions quickly. It is compressible when dry and expandable when wet and has high tensile strength, good elongation, and excellent resistance to most chemicals. PVA sponge is hydrophilic and can hold up to 12 times its dry weight in water. Cell size can be varied depending on the required use; the finer the cell, the better the capillary action. The wet sponge can withstand temperatures approaching 70°C and the dry about 100°C. PVA sponge is effectively inert and will not, in itself, support microbial growth. Extremely soft when wet, air-foaming soft cleaning PVA surgical sponges are hypoallergenic, which are suitable and ideal for soft and sensitive skin, specific in the use of surgical treatments such as carpal tunnel syndrome treatments via minimally invasive surgery.

Air-foaming soft cleaning PVA sponge with interlinked cell structure is perfect for any application where absorbency, durability, and versatility are key points. Air-foaming soft cleaning PVA requires different handling and processing than other more widely used foams. Strong chemical and abrasion resistance of air-foaming soft cleaning PVA sponges go through stringent quality control and super cleaning medical grade Cenefom PVA raw materials prepared in medical and clean room environments. Because of biocompatible properties, air-foaming soft cleaning

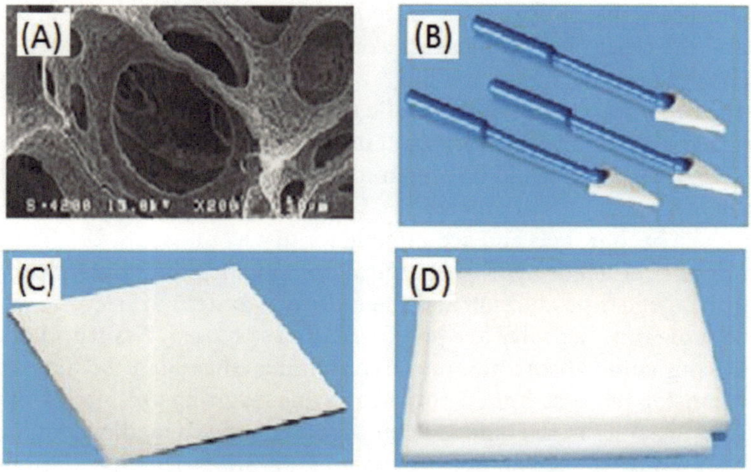

Figure 6.
The designed assistive dressings of air-foaming soft cleaning surgical sponge for carpal tunnel syndrome treatments via minimally invasive surgery (Medical grade Cenefom PVA foam in PARSD Pharmaceutical Technology Co.). (A) The SEM photo of the surgical sponge with an open-cell microstructure, (B) the photo of the surgical swab, (C) the photo of the dried surgical sponge, and (D) the photo of the wet surgical sponge.

PVA sponges were documented as being used for medical purposes. Available in a wide range of pore sizes and water-holding capacity could be selected for different clinical purposes (**Figure 6**). Furthermore, air-foaming soft cleaning PVA sponge and thin membrane provide strong chemical and abrasion resistance, non-linting, non-abrasive, latex Free, non-phthalate, biocompatible, UV resistant, withstanding temperatures of up to 70°C when wet and 100°C dry without deformation, extremely durable, available in a wide range of pore sizes.

3.4 Characterization of the assistive hydrogel surgical dressing with polymeric films designed for using after carpal tunnel syndrome treatments via minimally invasive surgery

Advanced dressings are designed to maintain a moist environment at the site of application, allowing the fluids to remain close to the wound but not spread to unaffected, healthy skin areas [25]. Several biomedical polymers are employed to be materials of hydrogel dressings such as polyvinyl alcohol, polymethacrylate, collagen, alginate, polyelectrolyte, water-soluble polymers, etc. [8–10, 14–16]. The relevance of the moist wound environment as a factor accelerating the healing process was first observed by Winter in 1962 but only recently has received more serious attention [26]. Dressings designed for moist wound healing are represented by hydrogel and hydrocolloid products. Both induce autolytic debridement, which facilitates the elimination of the dead tissue [27]. Hydrogel-based wound dressings are one of the most promising materials in wound care, fulfilling important dressing requirements, including keeping the wound moist while absorbing extensive exudate, adhesion-free coverage of sensitive underlying tissue, pain reduction of pain managements through cooling ability of hydrogel, and a potential for active intervention in the wound healing procedures [28, 29]. Because of the moisture provided to the wound from the moist hydrogel dressing with a moist swollen layer, common healing phases such as granulation, epidermis repair, and the removal of excess dead tissue become simplified. In addition to aiding the wound treatment stages, the cool sensation provided by the assistive hydrogel surgical dressing to the wound offers relief from pain for at least 6 hours. When hydration is provided for the wound bed, discomfort experienced from changing the dressing becomes reduced, and the risk of infection also becomes decreased. Hydrogels are widely used as debriding agents, moist dressings, and components of pastes for wound care because of the moist ability of amphiphilic materials and structures such as semi-interpenetrating polymeric networks and interpenetrating polymeric networks (IPN). The IPN structure could be prepared from multiple cross-linking reactions via thermal or photochemical procedures. However, they do not need further wound fluids to become gels and are suitable for dry wounds [28, 29]. The so-called "moisture donor" effect of hydrogel surgical dressing helps autolytic debridement, increasing collagenase production and the moisture content of necrotic wounds [25]. At the same time, a protective polymeric film was used. Assistive hydrogel surgical dressing could absorb and retain contaminated exudate within the gel mass through expansion of cross-linked polymer chains resulting in isolation of bacteria and detritus molecules in the liquid. Their high-water content allows vapor and oxygen transmission to the wounds such as pressure sores, leg ulcers, surgical and necrotic wounds, lacerations, and burns. Assistive hydrogel surgical dressing seems to play an important role as emergency burns treatment alone or in combination with other products, thanks to their cooling and hydrating effects [26]. Hence, the hydrogel surgical dressing with a polymeric film was designed for using after carpal tunnel syndrome treatments via minimally invasive surgery as shown in **Figure 7**.

3.5 LLLT for carpal tunnel syndrome treatments after minimally invasive surgery

Figure 7A shows a new design of optical guided medical device with LLLT sources and its key functional components for wound healing. Furthermore, **Figure 7B** shows clinical applications of new designed medical devices for carpal tunnel syndrome treatments via minimally invasive surgery and the wound healing of internal and

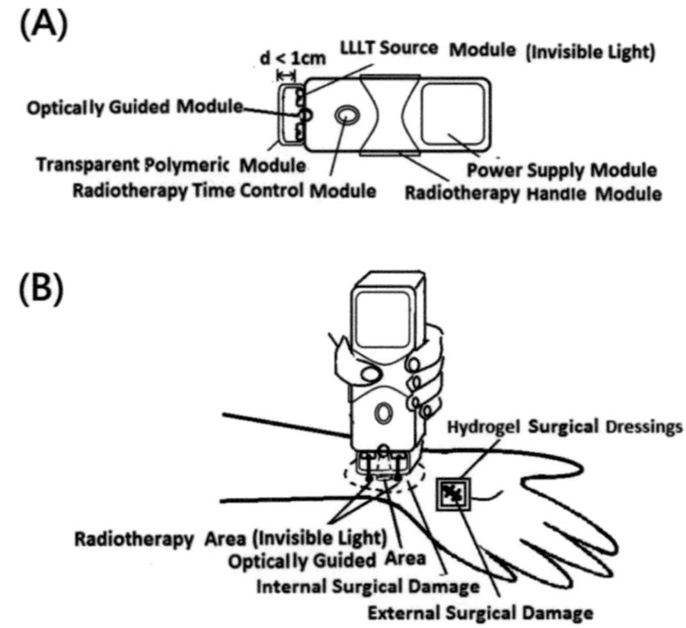

Figure 7.
(A) New design of optical guided medical device with LLLT sources for wound healing (Transverse Industries Co-design) and its key functional components. (B) Clinical applications of new designed medical devices for carpal tunnel syndrome treatments via MIS and the wound healing of internal and external surgical damages after elective surgery.

external surgical damage after elective surgery. Practically, a series of new designed medical devices with LLLT sources were employed for healing in internal and external surgical damages. Most important, the designed medical devices with LLLT sources were used for internal surgical damage such as the target ligament healing and reducing inflammation under the skin. The medical device with LLLT sources showed no damage H-bonding or molecule interaction. LLLT sources are not enough to change and damage cell or tissue molecule structure, have no remarkable increasing temperature (<0.1–0.5°C), and observed biological response being due to photobiostimulation. Most important, the designed medical devices with LLLT sources provide a kind of invasive immediately continuous treatments with no heat, no pain, no medicine, and no needle for internal surgical damage healing after MIS to greatly reduce the potential harms to the body and enhance convenience of healing wounds. LLLT, phototherapy, or photobiomodulation refers to the use of photons at a nonthermal irradiance to alter biological activity. LLLT uses coherent light sources (lasers), noncoherent light sources consisting of filtered lamps or LED, or laser, and, on occasion, a combination of both. The main medical applications of LLLT are reducing inflammation and pain and promoting regeneration of different tissues and nerves [30, 31]. In the past, laser therapies have been used increasingly for the esthetic treatment of fine wrinkles, aged skin, and scars, a process known as photo-rejuvenation (**Table 1**) [32]. Recently, this approach has also been used for inflammatory acne (**Table 1**) [32]. LLLT involves exposing cells or tissue to low levels of light sources. This process is referred to as "low level" because the energy or power densities used are low compared with other forms of laser therapy such as cutting or thermally coagulating tissue. More recently, clinical treatments with LLLT have been found to stimulate or inhibit an assortment of cellular processes or cellular photobiostimulation [33]. The basic biological mechanism would be thought to be through absorption of specific light by mitochondrial chromophores, in particular cytochrome *c* oxidase (CCO), which is contained in the respiratory chain located within the mitochondria [34–36], and perhaps also by photoacceptors

Supplier	Device name	Wavelength (nm)	Clinical applications
PhotoMedex (Manchester, UK)	OMNILUX	415(±5)/633(±6)/830(±5)	Acne, photodamage, nonmelanoma skin cancers, skin rejuvenation, vitiligo, and wound healing after elective surgery
OPUSMED (Montreal, Canada)	LumiPhase-R	660	Skin firmness, rhytid depth, and wrinkles
Lightwave technologies (Phoenix, AZ)	Lightwave professional deluxe LED system	630/880	Antiaging and skin rejuvenation
Dynatronics (Salt Lake City, UT)	Synergie LT12	660/880	Antiaging, skin firmness, wrinkles, skin tone, and texture for face and neck
Transverse (Taipei, TW)	TI-816	830/660	REHACARE, pain management, skin rejuvenation, wound healing after surgery, and nerve regeneration

Table 1.
The designed medical devices with different LLLT sources for relative clinical applications [30].

in the plasma membrane of cells. A cascade of events occurs consequently in the mitochondria, which leads to biostimulation of various systems in specific clinical applications (**Table 1**) [37]. Furthermore, absorption spectra obtained for cytochrome *c* oxidase in different oxidation states could be recorded and found to be similar to the action spectra for biological responses to the light [37]. The absorption of laser light energy could cause photodissociation of inhibitory nitric oxide (NO) from cytochrome *c* oxidase [38], leading to enhancement of enzyme activity [39], electron transport [40], mitochondrial respiration, and adenosine triphosphate production (**Table 1**) [41, 42]. LLLT is now used to treat a wide variety of ailments (**Table 1** and **Figure 7**) [30, 43–54]. In turn, LLLT alters the cellular redox state, which induces the activation of numerous intracellular signaling pathways, and alters the affinity of transcription factors concerned with cell proliferation, survival, tissue repair, and regeneration (**Table 1** and **Figure 7**) [34, 35, 44–54]. The medical devices with different LLLT sources are designed for relative clinical applications as listed in **Table 1**.

3.6 Clinical evaluation of carpal tunnel surgical procedure with the new designed medical devices

The clinical evaluation of carpal tunnel surgical procedures with the new light guided medical device was studied by a design of "clinical evaluation table of carpal tunnel surgical procedure." Also, three kinds of finger activities such as clenching, finger splaying, and touching from the index finger to thumb could be employed for clinical evaluation of carpal tunnel syndrome as shown in **Figure 8A–C**, respectively. Difficulty in the movement or coordination of the fingers in one or both hands hints possibility of carpal tunnel syndrome. It is because the median nerve would pass through the carpal tunnel to receive any kind of sensations from the thumb, index, and middle fingers of the hand. Numbness and tingling of the thumb, index, and the middle fingers in the hand are clinical evaluations for carpal tunnel syndrome by using three kinds of finger activities (**Figure 8**). The area of numbness and tingling of the thumb, index, and the middle fingers in the hand could be marked in the "clinical evaluation table of carpal tunnel surgical procedure" (**Table 2**). The red part involves the muscular dystrophy position of carpal tunnel syndrome as shown in **Table 2a**. The red marks of suture as shown in **Table 2b** indicate the cut position of carpal tunnel surgical procedure. Also, the "Suggesting Procedure before carpal tunnel surgical procedure" and "Suggesting Procedure after carpal tunnel surgical procedure" could be reported in the designed clinical evaluation table of "Carpal Tunnel Syndrome Treatments via minimally invasive surgery by using designed medical devices."

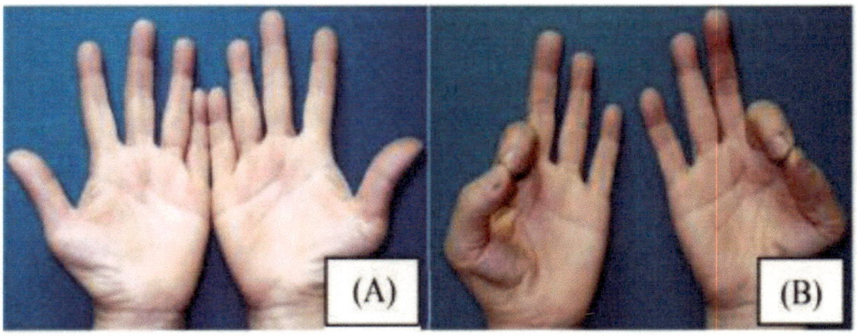

Figure 8.
Photos of two kinds of finger activities such as (A) finger splaying and (B) touching from the index finger to thumb for clinical evaluation of carpal tunnel syndrome [1].

DOI: http://dx.doi.org/10.5772/intechopen.82523

(a) Before carpal tunnel surgical procedure	**(b) After carpal tunnel surgical procedure**
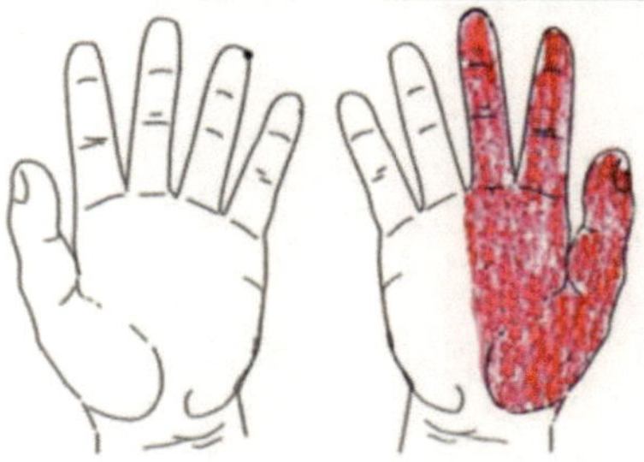	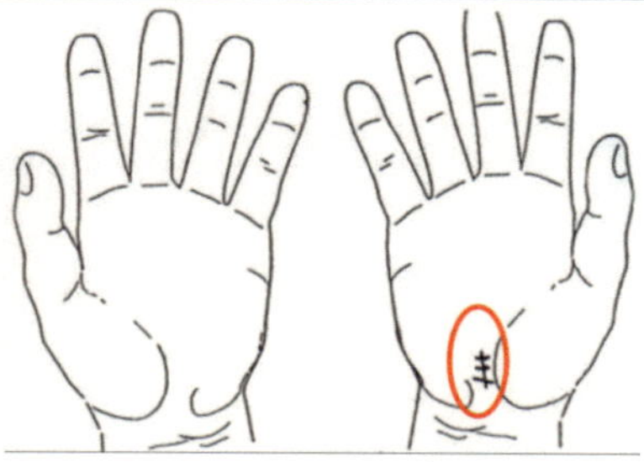
• Suggesting procedure: (*Date:* mm, dd, yyyy)	• Suggesting procedure: (*Date:* mm, dd, yyyy)
1. Carpal tunnel syndrome treatments via minimally invasive surgery	1. The wound healing of internal and external surgical damage after minimally invasive surgery 2. LLLT for internal surgical damages 3. The air-foaming soft cleaning surgical sponge for soft cleaning external surgical damages 4. The hydrogel surgical dressing for external surgical damages

Table 2.
The clinical evaluation table of "Carpal tunnel syndrome treatments via minimally invasive surgery by using designed medical devices" [1].

4. Summary

This study provides a novel design and fabrication of optical guided medical devices with a light scattering module for carpal tunnel syndrome. The LED light or laser could be employed as optical guided modules. A new medical device with optical LLLT module and a series of assistive surgical healing dressings such as air-foam soft cleaning sponges and hydrogel surgical dressings were also designed for wound healing in carpal tunnel syndrome treatments. Last, the designed medical devices such as optical guided medical devices and assistive surgical dressings could be found as a powerful device not only for carpal tunnel syndrome but also for related clinical applications.

Author details

Ching-Cheng Huang[1]* and Ming-Che Chiang[2]

1 Department of Biomedical Engineering, Ming-Chuan University, Taoyuan, Taiwan

2 Neurosurgery Department, Taichung Veterans General Hospital, Taichung, Taiwan

*Address all correspondence to: junas.tw@yahoo.com.tw

References

[1] Chiang MC, Huang CC. Biological and clinical evaluations of designed optically guided medical devices with scalpel and light scattering modules for carpal tunnel surgical procedure. Journal Bio-Medical Materials and Engineering (BMME). 2015;**26**:S173-S179

[2] Fu KL, Huang CC, Fu YC, Chiang MC. King-yard tech.: A safety surgical devices with bio-inspired trunk strengthening structure for minimally invasive surgery. Taiwan Patent 2018; M553983

[3] Fu KL, Huang CC, Fu YC, Chiang MC. King-Yard Tech.: A safety surgical devices with photo-guiding and positioning surgical modules for minimally invasive surgery. Taiwan Patent. 2017; M552335

[4] Liaw DJ, Huang CC, Sang HC, Wu PL. Macromolecular microstructure, reactivity ratio and viscometric studies of water-soluble cationic and/or Zwitterionic copolymers. Polymer. 2000;**41**:6123-6131

[5] Liaw DJ, Huang CC, Liaw BY. Synthesis and properties of polyurethanes based on bisphenol-S derivatives. Polymer. 1998;**39**:3529-3535

[6] Reddy TT, Kano A, Maruyama A, Hadano M, Takahara A. Thermosensitive transparent semi-interpenetrating polymer networks for wound dressing and cell adhesion control. Biomacromolecules. 2008;**9**(4):1313-1321

[7] Liaw DJ, Chen WH, Huang CC. Synthesis and characterization of new organosoluble poly(ether-imide)s derived from various novel bis (ether anhydride)s. In: Mittal KL, editor. Polyimides and Other High Temperature Polymers, Utrecht. Vol. 2. VSP Publisher; 2003. pp. 47-70

[8] Zhai G, Toh SC, Tan WL, Kang ET, Neoh KG, Huang CC, et al. Poly(vinyliden e fluoride) with grafted Zwitterionic polymer side chains for electrolyte-responsive microfiltration membranes. Langmuir. 2003;**19**:7030-7037

[9] Liaw DJ, Huang CC, Sang HC, Kang ET. Photophysical and solution properties of naphthalene-labeled styrene/N, N-dimethyl maleimido propylammonium propane sulfonate copolymer. Langmuir. 1999;**15**:5204-5211

[10] Vlierberghe SV, Cnudde V, Dubruel P, Masschaele B, Cosijns A, Patric IDP, et al. Porous gelatin hydrogels: 1. Cryogenic formation and structure analysis. Biomacromolecules. 2007;**8**(2):331-337

[11] Liaw DJ, Chen TP, Huang CC. Self-assembly aggregation of highly stable co-polynorbornenes with amphiphilic architecture via ring-opening metathesis polymerization. Macromolecules. 2005;**38**:3533-3538

[12] Kumar M, Sanford KJ, Cuevas WA, Katharine MD, Collier D, Chow N. Designer protein-based performance materials. Biomacromolecules. 2006;**7**(9):2543-2551

[13] Katsumata T, Maitani M, Huang CC, Shiotsuki M, Masuda T. Synthesis and proper ties of various poly(diphenylacetylenes) containing tert-amine moieties. Polymer. 2008;**49**:2808-2816

[14] Hrynyk M, Martins-Green M, Barron AE, Neufeld RJ. Alginate-PEG sponge architecture and role in the design of insulin release dressings. Biomacromolecules. 2012;**13**(5):1478-1485

[15] Liaw DJ, Huang CC, Kang ET. Effect of architecture and environments on

polymeric molecular assemblies of novel amphiphilic diblock copolynorbornenes with narrow polydispersity via living ring-opening metathesis polymerization (ROMP). Journal of Polymer Science Part A: Polymer Chemistry. 2006;**44**:2901-2911

[16] Liaw DJ, Huang CC, Ju JY. Novel star-like multifunctional polymeric materials with predominant cis microstructures derived from α-norbornenyl macromonomer and stable macroinitiator via ring-opening metathesis polymerization and atom transfer radical polymerization. Journal of Polymer Science, Part A: Polymer Chemistry. 2006;**44**:3382-3392

[17] Karakasyan C, Legros M, Lack S, Brunel F, Maingault P, Ducouret G, et al. Cold gelation of alginates induced by monovalent cations. Biomacromolecules. 2010;**11**:2966-2975

[18] Liu HW, Chen CH, Tsai CL, Lin IH, Hsiue GH. Heterobifunctional poly (ethylene glycol)-tethered bone morphogenetic protein-2-stimulated bone marrow mesenchymal stromal cell differentiation and osteogenesis. Tissue Engineering. 2007;**13**(5):1113-1124

[19] Makino A, Kurosaki K, Ohmae M, Kobayashi S. Chitinase-catalyzed synthesis of alternatingly N-deacetylated chitin: A chitin–chitosan hybrid polysaccharide. Biomacromolecules. 2006;**7**:950-957

[20] Chaw JR, Liu HW, Shih YC, Huang CC. New designed nerve conduits with porous ionic cross-linked alginate/chitosan structure for nervous regeneration. Journal Bio-Medical Materials and Engineering(BMME). 2015;**26**:S95-S102

[21] Zhai G, Toh SC, Tan WL, Kang ET, Neoh KG, Huang CC, et al. Poly(vinylidene fluoride) with grafted Zwitterionic polymer side chains for electrolyte-responsive microfiltration membranes. Langmuir. 2003;**19**:7030-7037

[22] Zhai G, Yu WH, Kang, Neoh KG, Huang CC, Liaw DJ. Functionalization of hydrogen-terminated silicon with polybetaine brushes via surface-initiated reversible addition-fragmentation chain-transfer (RAFT) polymerization. Industrial and Engineering Chemistry Research. 2004;**43**:1673-1680

[23] Kang ET, Neoh KG, Chen W, Tan KL, Liaw DJ, Huang CC. Surface structures and adhesion characteristics of poly(tetrafluoroethylene) films after modification by graft copolymerization. Journal of Adhesion Science and Technology. 1996;**10**:725-743

[24] Li ZF, Kang ET, Neoh KG, Tan KL, Huang CC, Liaw DJ. Surface structures and adhesive-free adhesion characteristics of polyaniline films after modification by graft copolymerization. Macromolecules. 1997;**30**:3354-3362

[25] Stashak TS, Farstvedt E, Othic A. Update on wound dressings: Indications and best use. Clinical Techniques in Equine Practice. 2004;**3**:148-163

[26] Osti E, Osti F. Treatment of cutaneous burns with burnshield (hydrogel) and a semi-permeable adhesive film. Annals of Burns and Fire Disasters. 2004;**7**:137-141

[27] Turner TD. Hospital usage of absorbent dressings. The Pharmaceutical Journal. 1979;**222**:421-424

[28] Murphy PS, Evans GRD. Advances in wound healing: A review of current wound healing products. Plastic Surgery International. 2012:**2012**;190436

[29] Koehler J, Brandl FP, Goepferich AM. Fast and excellent healing of hydroxypropyl guar gum/poly(N,N-dimethyl acrylamide)

hydrogels. European Polymer Journal. 2018;**100**:1-11

[30] Avci P, Gupta A, Sadasivam M, Vecchio D, Pam Z, Pam N, Hamblin MR. Low-level laser (light) therapy (LLLT) in skin: Stimulating, healing, restoring. Seminars in Cutaneous Medicine and Surgery. 2003;**32**:41-52

[31] Gupta A, Avci P, Sadasivam M. Shining light on nanotechnology to help repair and regeneration. Biotechnology Advances. 2013;**31**:607-631

[32] Seaton ED, Mouser PE, Charakida A. Investigation of the mechanism of action of nonablative pulsed-dye laser therapy in photorejuvenation and inflammatory acne vulgaris. The British Journal of Dermatology. 2006;**155**:748-755

[33] Barolet D. Light-emitting diodes (LEDs) in dermatology. Seminars in Cutaneous Medicine and Surgery. 2008;**27**:227-238

[34] Karu TI, Kolyakov SF. Exact action spectra for cellular responses relevant to phototherapy. Photomedicine and Laser Surgery. 2005;**23**:355-361

[35] Greco M, Guida G, Perlino E. Increase in RNA and protein synthesis by mitochondria irradiated with helium-neon laser. Biochemical and Biophysical Research Communications. 1989;**163**:1428-1434

[36] Karu TI, Pyatibrat LV, Kalendo GS. Photobiological modulation of cell attachment via cytochrome c oxidase. Photochemical & Photobiological Sciences. 2004;**3**:211-216

[37] Oron U. Light therapy and stem cells: A therapeutic intervention of the future? Interventional Cardiology. 2011;**3**(6):627-629

[38] Lane N. Cell biology: Power games. Nature. 2006;**443**:901-903

[39] Wong-Riley MT, Liang HL, Eells JT. Photobiomodulation directly benefits primary neurons functionally inactivated by toxins: Role of cytochrome c oxidase. Journal of Biological Chemistry. 2005;**280**:4761-4771

[40] Pastore D, Greco M, Petragallo VA. Increase in H+/e-ratio of the cytochrome c oxidase reaction in mitochondria irradiated with helium-neon laser. Biochemistry and Molecular Biology International. 1994;**34**:817-826

[41] Karu T, Pyatibrat L, Kalendo G. Irradiation with He-Ne laser increases ATP level in cells cultivated in vitro. Journal of Photochemistry and Photobiology. B. 1995;**27**:219-223

[42] Harris DM. Editorial comment biomolecular mechanisms of laser biostimulation. Journal of Clinical Laser Medicine & Surgery. 1991;**9**:277-280

[43] Liu H, Colavitti R, Rovira II. Redox-dependent transcriptional regulation. Circulation Research. 2005;**97**:967-974

[44] Peplow PV, Chung TY, Ryan B. Laser photobiomodulation of gene expression and release of growth factors and cytokines from cells in culture: A review of human and animal studies. Photomedicine and Laser Surgery. 2011;**29**:285-304

[45] Wang CZ, Chen YJ, Wang YH, Yeh ML, Huang MH, Ho ML, et al. Low-level laser irradiation improves functional recovery and nerve regeneration in sciatic nerve crush rat injury model. PLoS One. 2014;**9**(8):e103348

[46] Wu JY, Wang YH, Wang GJ, Ho ML, Wang CZ, Yeh ML, et al. Low-power GaAlAs laser irradiation promotes the proliferation and osteogenic differentiation of stem cells via IGF1 and BMP2. PLoS One. 2012;**7**(9):e044027

[47] Sculean A, Schwarz F, Becker J. Anti-infective therapy with an Er:YAG laser: Influence on peri-implant healing. Expert Review of Medical Devices. 2005;**2**(3):267-276

[48] Stadler I. In vitro effects of low level laser irradiation at 660 nm on peripheral blood lymphocytes. Lasers in Surgery and Medicine. 2000;**27**(3):255-261

[49] Karu TI. Mechanisms of low-power laser light action on cellular level. In: Simunovic Z, editor. Lasers in Medicine and Dentistry. Rijeka: Vitgraph; 2000. pp. 97-125

[50] Whelan HT, Smits RL, Buchman EV. Effect of NASA light emitting diode irradiation on wound healing. Journal of Clinical Laser Medicine & Surgery. 2001;**19**(6):305-314

[51] Rochkind S, Shahar A, Nevo Z. An innovative approach to induce regeneration and the repair of spinal cord injury. Laser Therapy. 1997;**9**(4):151

[52] Macedo AB, Moraes LHR, Mizobuti DS, Fogaca AR, Moraes FSR, Hermes TA, et al. Low-level laser therapy (LLLT) in dystrophin-deficient muscle cells: Effects on regeneration capacity, inflammation response and oxidative stress. PLoS One. 2015;**10**(6):e0128567

[53] Almeida-Lopes L. Comparison of the low level laser therapy effects on cultured human gingival fibroblasts proliferation using different irradiance and same fluence. Lasers in Surgery and Medicine. 2001;**29**(2):179-184

[54] Shefer G. Low energy laser irradiation promotes the survival and cell cycle entry of skeletal muscle satellite cells. Journal of Cell Science. 2002;**115**:1461-1469

Section 2

Peripheral Nerve Injury, Diagnosis and Treatment

Chapter 6

Biomaterials and Cellular Systems at the Forefront of Peripheral Nerve Regeneration

Rui Damásio Alvites, Mariana Vieira Branquinho, Ana Rita Caseiro, Sílvia Santos Pedrosa, Ana Lúcia Luís, Stefano Geuna, Artur Severo Proença Varejão and Ana Colette Maurício

Abstract

Peripheral nerve injuries remain a common clinical complication, and currently available therapies present significant limitations, often resulting in poor and suboptimal outcomes. Despite significant developments in microsurgical approaches in the last decades, no effective treatment options have been disclosed. Current research focuses on the optimization of such microsurgical techniques and on their combination with other pro-regenerative factors, such as mesenchymal stem cells or biomaterials. Mesenchymal stem cells present a remarkable capacity for bioactive molecule production that modulates inflammatory and regenerative processes, stimulating peripheral nerve regeneration. In parallel, efforts have been directed towards the development of biomaterial nerve guidance channels and nerve conduits. These biomaterials have been optimized in terms of biodegradability, ability to release bioactive factors, incorporation of cellular agents, and internal matrix architecture (to enable cellular migration and mimic native tissue morphology and to generate and bear specific electrical activity). The current literature review presents relevant advances in the development of mesenchymal stem cell and biomaterial-based therapeutic approaches aiming at the peripheral nerve tissue regeneration in diverse lesion scenarios, also exploring the advances achieved by our research group in this field in recent years.

Keywords: peripheral nerve injuries, nerve regeneration, cell-based therapies, biomaterials, animal models

1. Introduction

Peripheral nerve injuries result in temporary or permanent interruption of the connection between the nervous system and the effector organ, a phenomena defined as denervation, leading to functional changes and, ultimately, atrophic events [1]. These injuries bear significant impact to patients' health and well-being at both functional/physiological and psychological levels [2]. The negative impact of such morbidities is not limited to human individuals, and veterinary patients often present with comparable morbidities, contributing to the increased demand for improved therapeutic techniques [3]. Severe traumatic events (such as falls, road, or occupational accidents) result in the involvement of peripheral nerve structures in about 1–3% of the cases [3, 4]. Peripheral nerve affections may also present secondary to medical procedures such as surgeries, chemotherapy [5], and radiotherapy [6] or occur in consequence of chronic conditions such as neoplastic or metabolic diseases [7–9].

1.1 General anatomical features of the peripheral nerve

Peripheral nerve structures are composed of motor, sensory, and sympathetic fibers, forming specific nerve types that enervate the effector organs or sensory endings after emerging from the central nervous system (spinal cord) [10]. The cell bodies of sensory neurons are found in the dorsal root ganglia located in the intervertebral foramina, proximal to the site of fusion with the ventral roots. In the case of motor neurons, the cell body is situated in the central nervous system (CNS), more specifically in the anterior horns of the gray matter [11]. The nerve fiber is the functional unit of each nerve, consisting of axons and Schwann cells. Schwann cells are glial cells that are located longitudinally to the axons, of either myelinated or unmyelinated nerve fibers [10]. In the peripheral nerve, fibers of different diameters coexist, but only fibers with larger diameters are coated with a myelin sheath. In these cases, the Schwann cell wraps the axon segment concentrically. The small areas between two Schwann cells are called nodes of Ranvier, which enable the ionic exchange between the axon's axoplasm and the intercellular space and the saltatory conduction of the nerve impulse. The "jumps" of the impulses between the different nodes of Ranvier accelerate signal conduction. The fibers with smaller diameters appear grouped, and, although enveloped by the Schwann cell membrane, they are not coated by a myelin sheath. Thus, these fibers do not have the necessary structure for saltatory conduction, and the transmission of impulses along the axons is slower. Besides the myelin production, Schwann cells and their basal membrane structurally orient the axons and are sources of trophic and growth factors, ensuring the maintenance of the neighboring axons [10, 12].

The peripheral nerves are lined by three layers of connective tissue. Each axon is directly involved by the *endoneurium*, a matrix of longitudinal collagen fibers of small diameter associated with a thin network of microvessels. It grants little mechanical protection, and the capillary network acts as blood-nerve barrier [13]. Within the endoneurial layer, there are myelinated or non-myelinated fibers in association with the Schwann cells. A nervous fascicle is a set of axons covered by *endoneurium*, and the interfascicular endoneurium is the supporting framework for the nerve fibers. Nerve fasciculi may vary in number and size, depending on the nerve and the more proximal or distal anatomical position. Each nerve fascicle is further coated with a layer of consistent connective tissue called *perineurium*. *Perineurium* comprises a set of collagen fibrils of oblique, circular, and longitudinal orientation, constituted by two lamellae, working as a diffusion barrier. The outer lamella presents endocytic vesicles responsible for molecular transport. The inner lamella has tight junctions between adjacent perineurial cells, regulating the transport of macromolecules and contributing to the maintenance of the blood-nerve barrier. The *perineurium* is the greatest mechanical protection against tensile forces [14, 15]. The entire nerve trunk is further covered by a final layer of connective tissue, named *epineurium*, representing about half of the total diameter of the peripheral nerve. In some locations, the *epineurium* extends internally and separates directly the nerve fascicles (*interfascicular epineurium*). The internal portion of the *epineurium* has its own network of blood vessels and varying amounts of fat tissue. The external portion, enveloping the entire nerve, defines its anatomical shape. Although the *epineurium* contributes to protection against tensile forces, it does not form specific barriers [16]. The blood supply of the peripheral nerves is achieved through the small vessels of the *epineurium*, *perineurium*, and *endoneurium*. This intrinsic blood supply system presents particular features, such as endothelial tight junctions that aid in the diffusion of compounds. Thus, this intrinsic vascular network is crucial during nerve regeneration, as the blood-nerve barrier modulates its function after the injury, allowing the flow of growth factors, immune cells, and other macromolecules into the endoneurial space [17]. The extrinsic blood supply component consists of blood vessels with different diameter that originate from larger arteries and veins in the vicinity of the nerve. Once these vessels reach the *epineurium*, they branch out, and their ascending and descending branches supply the intraneural plexuses [10].

1.2 Peripheral nerve lesions and their functional consequences

The most common type of peripheral nerve injuries are those resulting from transections (usually because of penetrating traumas), over-stretching, and compression. The effects of nerve compression are reversible when the aggression is sustained for a short period [18]. Other lesions include those caused by lacerations and ischemia [2]. Primary nerve affections originate from a force directly applied to the nerve tissue, with secondary lesions developing from the vascular and ischemic damages. Peripheral nerves have notable inherent malleability due to their collagen content. When this adaptation threshold is exceeded, the lesion occurs [19]. For example, the small arteries responsible for blood irrigation of the peripheral nerves can be compressed by hematomas developed secondarily to the initial lesion, with subsequent restriction in blood supply [20]. The main consequences are motor, sensory, and autonomic functional disturbances and deficits in the body segments that undergo denervation [21].

Seddon introduced a grading system for PNI, initially considering three levels of injury: neuropraxia, axonotmesis, and neurotmesis [22]. Later, Sunderland expanded the system to five categories, with grades 1 and 5 corresponding to neuropraxia and neurotmesis, respectively, and grades 2–4 corresponding to subdivisions of axonotmesis [23]. Grade 4 and 5 injuries are those that require surgical intervention/reconstruction. Although this classification system correlates with the histological image of specific injury models, most lesions are mixed and encompass two or more components. In 1988 a sixth mixed injury was added to the Sunderland system by Mackinnon and Dellon (**Table 1**) [24].

Peripheral nervous system (PNS) has a superior regenerative capacity when compared to the CNS [25], due to the intrinsic and functional characteristics of each system: while the cell body of the peripheral nerve is not often affected during the lesion, CNS damage frequently results in direct neuronal death. Concerning the PNS, the age of the patient, category of the injury, and integrity of the cell body directly influence the regenerative efficiency [26]. Most importantly, the regenerative efficiency relates to the time elapsed between the occurrence of the injury and the therapeutic intervention. This time frame influences speed of recovery of nerve structures, its function, and the capacity to respond to electrophysiological stimulation, which are all essential factors in the prevention of muscular atrophy and organ dysfunctions [27].

When therapeutic or surgical interventions are delayed, the activation of Schwann cells and their stimulation over axonal growth have been demonstrated to be less effective, and more severe degenerative phenomena are observed [28, 29].

Grade	Characteristics	Functional consequences
I	• **Neuropraxia** • Compressive or slight crush lesions; • Schwann cell are affected, with occurrence of focal demyelination; • Wallerian degeneration rarely occurs; • The integrity and continuity of axons and connective tissue are maintained; • Occurrence of nerve conduction blocks;	• Temporary paralysis of affected body segments; • Muscle atrophy is rare; • Rearrangement of the myelin sheath within 3 to 4 weeks and recovery within days to weeks; • No need for surgical intervention;
II	• **Axonotmesis;** • Crushing and stretching injuries; • Disruption of the axon and its myelin coating; • Basal lamina, *Endoneurium*, *perineurium* and *epineurium* are intact, with maintenance of the nerve's anatomical shape; • Occurrence of Wallerian degeneration distal to the lesion site;	• Good recovery rate, the reorganization taking months but depending on the level of structural disorder and the distance to the effector organ; • Partial lesions of the *endoneurium* may occur, directly affecting the prognosis; • Rarely requires surgical intervention;
III	• Crushing and stretching injuries; • Disruptive lesion of the axon, its myelin coating and *endoneurium*; • Occurrence of Wallerian degeneration distal to the lesion site; • Intact *perineurium* and *epineurium*, with maintenance of the nerve's anatomical shape.	• Recovery can occur over several months with conservative treatment, and can be speed up if the entrapment sites that hinder the regenerative sequence are released with surgical procedures; • Misdirection of regenerating axons may occur, with development of unrecoverable functional deficits.
IV	• Crushing and stretching injuries; • Disruptive lesion of the axon, its myelin coating, *endoneurium* and *perineurium*; • Intact *epineurium*;	• Occurrence of intranerve hemorrhage and presence of fibrous tissue leads to fascicular discontinuity, with consequent imprisonment of axonal buds, delay or hindrance of its growth. • Development of neuromas in continuity is common; • Surgical intervention required;
V	• **Neurotmesis;** • Pungent injuries, destructive forces and local administration of toxic products; • Complete transection of the nerve, with disruption of the axons, all its coating layers and disconnection between the proximal and distal segments.	• Total loss of function; • The absence of collagen coating layers interferes with the axonal regrowth and the normal regenerative sequence; • Development of neuromas on the separated nerve stumps; • Spontaneous recovery is impossible; • Surgical intervention required;
VI	• **Mixed lesion;** • Common in penetrating trauma and fractures near peripheral nerves;	• Recovery and necessity of therapeutic and surgical intervention depends on the type of injury and respective degrees of severity;

Table 1.
Peripheral nerve injury grading system and respective characteristics.

Likewise, muscles and effector organs that do not receive nervous stimuli during long periods suffer more serious structural and contractile changes, and the recovery of electrical communication becomes increasingly difficult to achieve [28].

1.3 Wallerian degeneration, endogenous regeneration, and response to nerve damage

The regenerative process is preceded by an initial physiological degenerative phase [30]. Immediately after the PNI (**Figure 1a**), a complex local response is established, involving both the axon segments of the injured nerve and the surrounding non-neural cells. With no communication with the neuron's cell body, the distal axonal segment maintains the ability to transmit electrical impulses for 48–96 h after injury. However, the swelling of the axonal end occurs within few hours after injury, due to the accumulation of lysosomes and axoplasmatic organelles in the paranodal regions that cannot progress beyond the site of injury. These events incur in the stretching and thinning of adjacent myelin sheaths (**Figure 1b**). After 12–24 h, the axonal microtubules disorganize, and the dissolution of the axonal skeleton begins. In the first or second days after injury, an influx of calcium ions activates

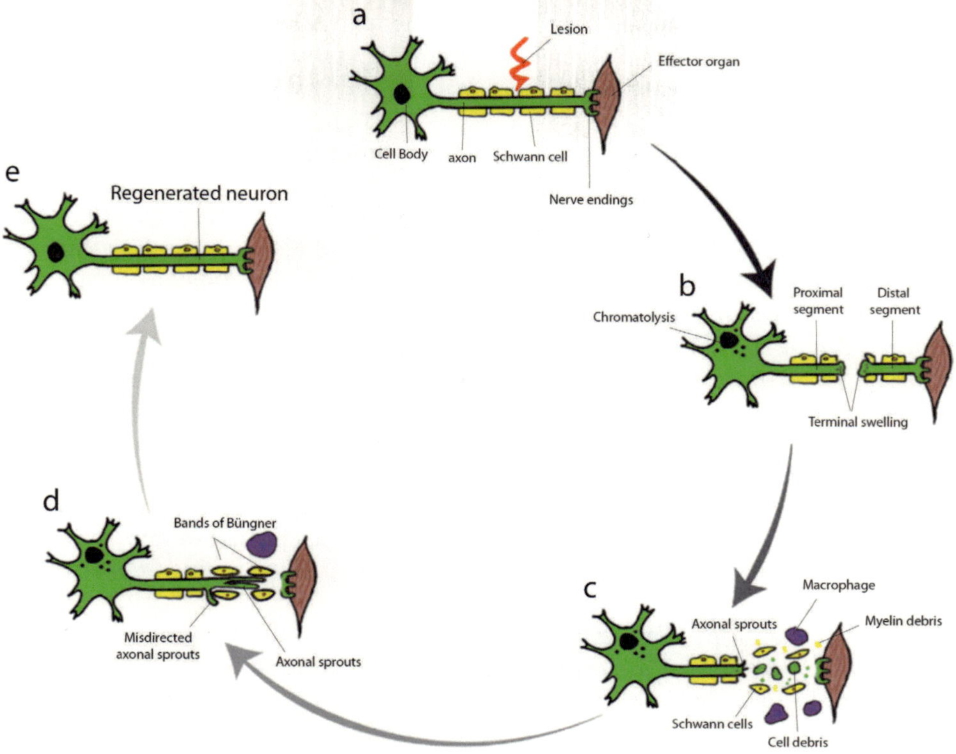

Figure 1.
Schematic representation of degeneration and regeneration of the peripheral nerve after injury: (a) PNI. (b) Chromatolysis and terminal swelling in the proximal and distal axonal segments. (c) Degradation of axons and myelin with release of debris. Cell and myelin debris are phagocytosed by macrophages and Schwann cells. Axonal sprouts are formed. (d) The axonal sprouts grow with the support of the bands of Büngner. The remaining macrophages undergo apoptosis or return to circulation. (e) Regenerated neuron.

calcium-dependent calpain proteins, which degrade axonal neurofilaments, releasing granular debris (granular disintegration) (**Figure 1c**) [31].

Within few minutes of lesion, the Schwann cells promote the degeneration of the myelin sheaths associated with the distal segment. After 24–36 h, changes become evident throughout the distal segment, with swelling of Schwann cells, compressing the associated axons. Myelin destruction is installed within 48 h after injury, which is fragmented into ovoid structures by the digestive chambers present in the cytoplasm of Schwann cells. An identical process is observed on unmyelinated Schwann cells, minus the fragmentation of the myelin [32]. Axonal and myelin fragments are then eliminated by cells with phagocytic capacity (macrophages and other myelomonocytic cells) and by the Schwann cells themselves (**Figure 1c**) [33]. The production and release of interleukins by these cells activates and stimulates the activity of other Schwann cells and fibroblastic populations [34, 35]. Once clearance of all axonal and myelin debris occurs, macrophages are eliminated by local apoptosis or by reentering in circulation.

Simultaneously, the mitotically quiescent Schwann cells are activated and proliferate within their original basal lamina, organizing themselves to create longitudinally oriented structures. These structures are called bands of Büngner and are important in the next phase of nerve regeneration, providing biochemical and structural support to the new axonal sprouts as they proliferate (**Figure 1d**) [36].

After the degeneration phase, the regeneration begins, which can be successfully concluded or abortive. The proximal segment undergoes an initial degeneration phase up to the last preserved internode in an identical manner to that occurring in the distal segment but of smaller extension. The most important phenomenon of the proximal segment is chromatolysis, while genetic upregulation and downregulation are established, metabolically preparing cells for the next phase (**Figure 1b**) [35, 37].

In the first 24 h after the injury, many axonal sprouts protrude from the most distal node of Ranvier of the proximal segment and bulge into a growth cone rich in metabolically active organelles. The progression of these sprouts is guided by the bands of Büngner [38], which are indispensable for guiding the expanding axons and secrete neurotrophic and transcription factors, creating a conducive environment to the growth of axonal buds [29]. Proteases are also released from the growth cone to degrade the fibrous, hemorrhagic, or inflammatory tissues and facilitate the progression of the axonal sprouts [39]. Only a few of the axonal extensions will contact the receptor at the distal ends (**Figure 1d**). In theory, an increased number of axonal sprouts reaching the target segment correspond to more extensive and effective neural regeneration (**Figure 1e**). The axonal extensions that do not reach the distal segment are eliminated to prevent misdirected and disorganized growth and possible development of neuromas. Nevertheless, occurrence of misdirected or erroneous axonal growth and its subsequent ineffective innervation of target tissues is often observed [40].

The quality and speed of nerve regeneration is improved when occurring in a well-vascularized site and in the presence of small amounts of scar tissue. Besides mechanical factors, the time elapsed between injury and complete repair and its functional recuperation prognosis depend on factors such as the age of the patient, the type of nerve, the site of the nerve that was injured, the cause of the injury and effect on neighboring tissues resulting from the injury [1, 2, 41, 42]. Nonetheless, even when endogenous repair mechanisms are effective, regenerated nerves often present thinner myelin sheets and shorter nodal lengths and result in functional deficits [43].

1.4 Therapeutic options for peripheral nerve injury

There are several therapeutic options available to address PNI, ranging from conservative to surgical approaches. Despite all efforts and advances achieved in recent years towards the effective repair of peripheral nerve after injury, the ultimate outcomes are still far from ideal, and recovery rates remain limited.

The success of any therapy prospected for the application in PNI will depend on the acceleration of the axonal regeneration rate achieved and modulation of the local microenvironment, therefore impacting on the chronicity of installed denervation and established consequences in the effector organs [44]. Thus, even if initial immobilization with physical therapy may be considered in some cases to ensure patient comfort, quick surgical reconstruction, associated or not to other therapeutic options, should be favored to promote improved nerve regeneration (**Figure 2**).

The primary repair of the injured nerve resourcing to microsurgical techniques is the recommended approach in case of neurotmesis lesion. To get the desired results, however, the expected success in peripheral nerve structure and function depends on the timing of reconstruction, and the intervention must be performed within a short period after the occurrence of the lesion. Epineural repair is one of such techniques, employed when tension-free coaptation of the nerve margins is possible within a well-vascularized local microenvironment [45]. In the first phase of the surgical technique, the injured nerve endings are intervened to remove necrotic tissue, cells, and inflammatory debris (originating from neurolysis), exposing the viable nerve stumps. In the subsequent phase, the two nerve tops

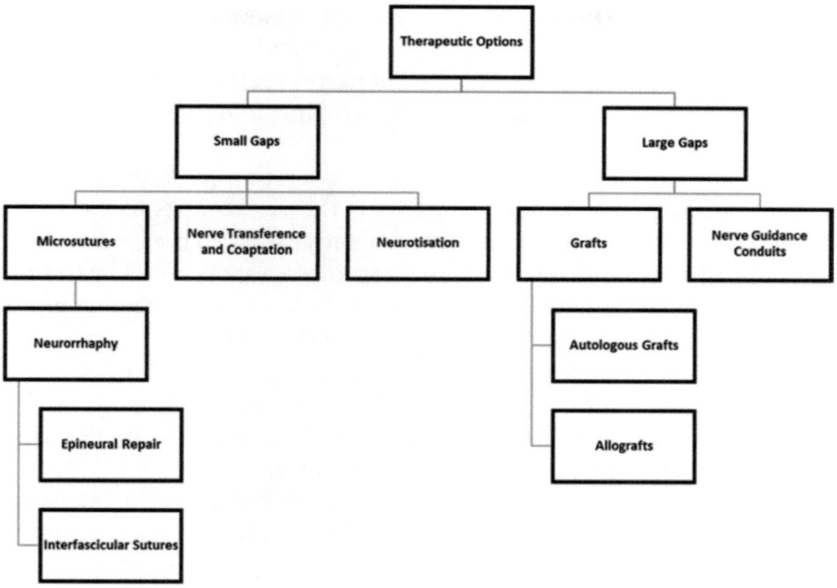

Figure 2.
Schematic representation of therapeutic options for PNI treatment.

are re-approached and anatomically coapted to achieve a minimum gap between them. This small space is quickly filled in with blood, phagocytes, and a fibrin matrix and plays a critical role in the transportation of Schwann cells between the two segments of injured nerves. Perfect coaptation between the two nerve ends is achieved through the application of interrupted micro sutures (neurorrhaphy) in the *epineurium*, aiming at the maintenance of the physiological position of the nerve segments, avoiding relative rotation displacement [46]. In larger nerve structures, the application of a micro suture between nerve fascicles of the two nerve segments after a careful intranerve dissection may be necessary. Theoretically, this technique sustains better fascicular alignment, but the trauma resulting from the extended dissection and the exuberant scarring phenomena resulting from the presence of the suture embedded in the nerve structure entail undesired side effects, precluding the success of this nerve reconstruction technique [47]. When direct neurorrhaphy is not possible [48, 49], an alternative technique includes the connection between the proximal segment of a nearby healthy nerve and the distal segment of the injured one (neurotization). A reimplantation when nerve root avulsion occurs is also possible [50].

When the injury results in nerve tissue loss and a gap forms between the two nerve segments, grafting techniques may be used to bridge the tissue gap and guide the regenerating axons in a tension-free manner [51]. Nevertheless, grafting techniques are not devoid of disadvantages [51, 52]. Autologous nerve grafts are one of the described options, due to the microstructural composition that facilitates axonal migration and the decreased risk of immune rejection reactions at the grafting site. However, this technique requires the sacrifice of a healthy nerve with proper dimensions and diameter, which is a limiting factor to its widespread application [53]. Allogeneic grafts are a complementary option, generally collected from cadaveric donors. Despite retaining the tissular microstructures, the risk of rejection at the receptor site increases, and concomitant immunosuppressive treatments are required [54]. These allografts can be decellularized through enzymatic treatment, minimizing the risk of inflammatory reaction and reducing the necessity for immunosuppression, improving their success rate [55].

Nerve sheets have also been used to promote the reparation of diverse injured tissues and in the promotion of nerve recovery after PNI, stimulating an early restitution of vascularization. The nerve sheet plays a scaffold function without promoting immunogenic reactions, ensuring cytokines and growth factors that stimulate axonal survival and regrowth [56, 57].

The use of nerve guidance conduits (NGCs), in a technique known as entubulation or tubulization, presents as an alternative to the use of grafts. These conduits provide physical separation between the regenerative site and the neighboring reactive (fibrous) tissue, preserving the neurogenic factors secreted by the injured nerve terminations [58–60]. The NGCs are described to outperform organic grafts in small nerve reconstruction [55], but the general lack of internal microstructural characteristics limits their application in the bridging of small nerve gaps [61, 62], particularly when not combined with cell-based therapies or locally applied growth factors (**Figure 3**). Therefore, NGCs function mostly as structural guides to promote the alignment of the two nerve ends, while the repair process of the nerve gap itself is promoted by the complementary therapies applied [63]. The biomaterials deemed adequate to shape the NGCs are expected to comply with a set of criteria that guarantee their safety and efficacy, as listed:

- Biocompatibility with target tissue (not triggering local or systemic inflammatory or organic rejection responses) [64]
- Absence of toxicity
- Biodegradability [65]
- Mechanical and structural stability during the regenerative process [66]
- Mechanical resistance to application of sutures and to the occurrence of mild local inflammatory reactions [66]
- Balanced flexibility and resistance to avoid compression of the nervous tissue during the reparation and to attenuate the hoarding of fibrous tissue and inflammatory secretions within the NGCs [67]
- Selective porosity and permeability (avoiding excessive loss of neurotrophic factors, tolerating entry of nutrients and oxygen, while controlling inflammatory cell influx to the injury site) [59, 68]
- Capacity to direct axonal growth distally [69]
- Adequate technical production, sterilizations, storing, and manipulation procedures [70]

The selection of the most suited biomaterial must also address the required dimensions and wall thickness required for the proper alignment and connection between the two nerve ends, without tension or compression, factors that may influence the rate of regeneration [71]. Diverse materials have been described, from natural and synthetic resorbable to non-resorbable devices. Regardless of the selected option, the ideal biomaterial must be capable of protecting the nerve tissue, avoid the development of neuromas, diminish the occurrence of tissue adhesions, guarantee a negligible inflammatory response, and stimulate regeneration of the axon [72].

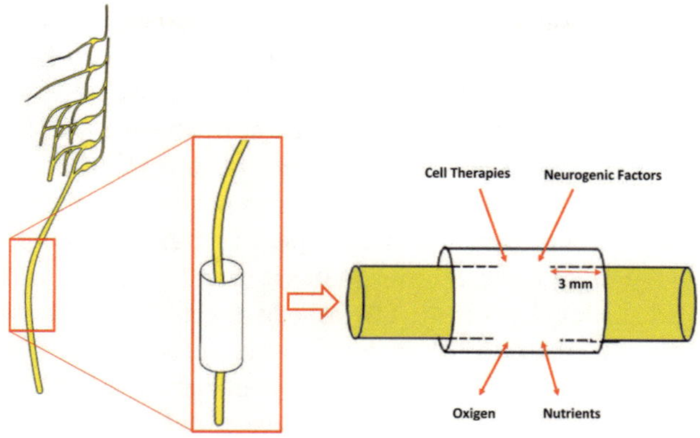

Figure 3.
Schematic representation of the application of an NGC in the rat sciatic nerve.

Although biomaterials alone can withstand, guide, and, in some extent, reestablish the continuity of the injured axons, the effectiveness of this entire process remains globally limited, particularly if longer gaps are considered [62]. In the current therapeutic scenario, the true advantages of using biomaterials reside in their combined use with cellular systems and neurotrophic factors [73]. Neurotrophic factors or neutrophins are produced and released naturally during the nerve regeneration process. These can be secreted by neuronal or non-neuronal cells, at both nerve ends, and are essential to conduct the regenerative sequence. Its function is mainly to stimulate neural differentiation and guide axonal growth [74]. Although these factors can be directly administered to the injured nerve, their application inside the lumen or on the wall of the NGCs (allowing a continuous release by diffusion into the lesion) presents as a more effective technique in longer nerve gaps. Without NGC support, the neurotrophic factors may diffuse freely towards neighboring tissues, deviating from the injury site, failing to support the regenerative process [57]. Different neurogenic factors have been proposed in studies on axonal regeneration, including glial cell-derived neurotrophic factor (GDNF); neuregulin-1, superfamily growth factor beta; brain-derived neurotrophic factor (BDNF); neurotrophins 3, 4, and 5; insulin-like growth factors; nerve growth factor (NGF); ciliary neurotrophic factor; and a combination of several factors such as platelet-rich plasma [75, 76].

Regenerative therapies based on the use of cellular agents are a promise to improve the therapeutic efficacy of techniques developed to stimulate peripheral nerve regeneration. Embryonic stem cells are theoretically the most versatile regenerative population, but their affective applicability for clinical purposes remains a contradictory topic, mostly due to the extreme ethical issues associated [77]. In the regenerative processes, native to the peripheral nerve, the Schwann cells represent a crucial regulatory role and therefore have been proposed as regenerative enablers. However, important limitations envisioning their clinical application have been noted, such as the associated donor site morbidity, the challenging ex vivo culturing and expansion protocols, and the complex therapeutic application. In addition, Schwann cells' availability is age-dependent (decreasing with the increasing age of the donor) [78].

In recent years, interest in the use of mesenchymal stem cells (MSCs) has increased significantly, particularly because of their assigned aptitude for cell and tissue differentiation and their capacity to adapt to each site of injury and to produce growth factors related to reparative phenomena. Also, they locally and systemically modulate the inflammatory reactions [79]. MSCs can be isolated from virtually all tissues on the organism (niches), such as the dental pulp, the synovial membrane, the olfactory mucosa, the placenta, and the umbilical cord Wharton's jelly [80–83]. To be classified as "true" MSCs, these cells have to manifest a set of specific characteristics: plastic adherence under standard culture conditions; lack of expression of hematopoietic markers (CD11b, CD14, CD34, CD45, CD79α, or CD19) as well as major histocompatibility complex II/human leukocyte antigen-DR; expression of the unspecific markers CD44, CD73, CD90, CD105; and capacity to, at least, trilineage in vitro differentiation (osteogenic, chondrogenic, and adipogenic) [84]. The ease of expansion of these populations, their capacity of differentiation in different cell lines, the tropism for lesion sites, their immunoprivileged phenotype, and capacity of trophic stimulation and modulation of tissue functions turn them into excellent candidates for therapeutic adjuvants [85]. Regarding the immunoprivileges of MSCs, these cells have long been referred as hypoimmunogenic, with the ability to cross most of the histocompatibility barriers without triggering an immune response [86]. However, some studies identified the production of antibodies against these populations and immune rejection after allogeneic donation, raising debate on this topic [87]. MSCs administered from allogeneic donations have been described to promote infiltration of macrophages and neutrophils at the injection site [88, 89] and to stimulate a donor- and dose-dependent blood-mediated inflammatory reaction [90]. There are also references to adverse clinical reactions following intra-articular administration of allogenic MSCs in the equine model [91, 92] and evidence of early death of MSCs after administration [93]. To fully understand the potential and limitations of allogeneic MSC therapies, deeper investigation is required on the immune response elicited and whether such responses may affect the therapeutic outcome.

In specific PNI scenarios, MSCs are described to intervene through several mechanisms, namely, secreting neurotrophic factors that stimulate neurogenesis and proliferation of Schwann cells; undergoing neurogenic or neuroglial (Schwann cells) differentiation; or modulating the local inflammatory response and the Wallerian degeneration [94]. The neurotrophic factors produced and secreted by MSCs include ciliary growth factors, neurotrophins, endothelial growth factors, glial-derived neurotrophic factors, NGF, and BDNF [29]. Remyelination of injured axons is also promoted by the MSCs since they can differentiate into cells presenting morphology and phenotypical markers of Schwann cells, becoming capable of promoting myelination [85, 95, 96].

Despite the prospected advantages, the optimum mode of administration of MSCs to the lesion site is still unclear. The simplest technique would be the microinjection of a cellular suspension at the injury site, but associated risks include trauma to resident cells and intraneural architecture and uneven cell distribution. The individual application of the MSCs, although being associated with improved outcomes, still denotes limited advantage over the traditional surgical techniques [97]. An alternative to the direct injection of the MSCs is their combination with a supporting matrix (such as fibrin) and their combined deposition at the lesion site [98]. Overall, the efficacy of MSCs is suggested to increase when in association with biomaterials (such as NGCs) and growth factors, granting increased success rate and functional recovery [99].

2. Biomaterials and peripheral nerve regeneration

Diverse biomaterials have been proposed in attempt to establish the best options to promote peripheral nerve regeneration after PNI.

2.1 Biological nerve conduits

Natural polymers, usually based on carbohydrates or proteins, are frequently applied as scaffolds to promote the regeneration of different tissues. Natural or biological biomaterials are described to easily stimulate cell adhesion, migration, proliferation, and growth. However, batch-to-batch variations of raw materials are often observed and limit the standardization of final product composition and manufacturing protocols [100].

2.1.1 Collagen

Collagen is seen by many researchers as the "perfect" material for regenerative medicine applications, since it is a major protein constituent in the extracellular matrix. Collagen has a regenerative effect on nerve tissue by transducing essential signals that stimulate cell adhesion, migration, proliferation, survival, and differentiation. Besides, it creates a supportive environment for connective tissues surrounding the blood vessels, ligaments, bone, cartilage, tendons, and skin, in both natural environment and regeneration sites. Collagen can be found and isolated from various animal tissue sources.

The advantageous characteristics of collagen include its physical resistance, low level of antigenicity, good biological compatibility, and the ability to be tailored and cross-linked, modulating water uptake and mechanical degradation rates. Of the 27 different types of collagen identified to date, the most abundant and widely investigated in biomedical engineering and regenerative medicine is the type I [101], which constitutes approximately 30% of mammalian musculoskeletal tissue [102]. For nerve regeneration, collagen type IV, a non-fibril forming collagen and the main component of the basement membrane, must also be considered due to its interaction with the Schwann cells [103]. Studies on the effectiveness of equine collagen type III have also been performed [104].

Collagen has been utilized as a scaffold, in the form of a gelatinous matrix, to stimulate neural regeneration, but it can also be processed in different formats of three-dimensional structures like gels, porous sponges, sheets [101], particles, and foams [105]. The application of collagen filaments (not organized in a conduit shape) promoted an effective guided axonal regeneration of 20 mm nerve defects [106], and NGCs containing a gel of collagen with Schwann cells were described to induce the growing of new neurites [107]. Collagen fibers within gels can be longitudinally aligned using magnetic fields and result in an improved neurite outgrowth when compared to that observed with randomly oriented collagen fibers [108]. Moreover, collagen NGCs containing a porous collagen glycosaminoglycan matrix promoted regeneration levels similar to those resulting from nerve autograft [109, 110]. Finally, commercial collagen type III membranes (commercially available as GentaFleece®, Baxter, Nuremberg, Germany) were demonstrated to promote the regeneration of rat sciatic nerves undergoing neurotmesis [104] and axonotmesis [111].

Various collagen-based conduits/devices are FDA-approved. In the process of manufacturing these NGCs, the matrix is molded tubularly while preserving the natural fibrillar characteristics of the collagen:

- NeuraGen® (approved in 2001) was demonstrated not to cause neuropathy by compression [112], a common observation when using rigid materials, and sustained nerve repair in the period of 4 weeks [110].

- NeuroMatrix™ and Neuroflex™ (both approved in 2001; Collagen Matrix, Inc., Franklin Lakes, NJ, USA) are flexible, resorbable, and non-friable NGCs that present a semipermeable tubular matrix, holding pores with diameters between 0.1 and 0.5 μm, thus allowing the transference of nutrients. Both nerve conduits are absorbed within 4–8 months after implantation, differ in the kink resistance, and are indicated for application in nerve defects smaller than 2.5 cm [68].

- NeuraWrap™ (2004; Integra LifeSciences Co), presenting the same constitution of NeuraGen®, is described to promote minimal scar tissue formation due to the porous outer membrane, capable of resisting compression by the neighboring tissue. Also, NeuraWrap™ promotes minimal nerve encapsulation and entrapment and avoids the formation of neuromas. Finally, it promotes an environment conducive to regeneration, because of a semipermeable inner membrane that allows the exchange and transport of nutrients [113].

- NeuroMend™ (2006; Collagen Matrix, Inc.) is a semipermeable device, designed so it can be unwound and spontaneously curl around the injured nerve, adapting perfectly to its shape and dimensions. The semipermeable membrane also allows the circulation of nutrients, regulating the movement of fibroblasts and inflammatory elements [114, 115].

Besides the available commercial nerve conduits, other studies describe the utilization of pure or blended collagen devices. Nerve conduits releasing neurotrophic factors such as GDNF and NGF were reported to result in improved reparation of nerve defects when compared with commercially available products such as Neurolac™ or NeuraGen® [57]. Micro-patterned tubular collagen matrices applied to the rat sciatic nerve model also demonstrated good pro-regenerative capacity [116]. In a work presented by Yang and Chen, the interaction between composite scaffolds obtained from blending a cross-linking chitosan with icariin and collagen revealed successful cell attachment, establishing the material as suitable for the support of cells in nerve regenerative therapies [117]. Cerri et al. compared the efficacy of collagen scaffolds with different porous microstructures in promoting sciatic nerve regeneration in the rat model of axonotmesis. A complete replacement of the conduit by normal nerve tissue was observed 60 days after injury, associated with a progressive regulation of genes and myelination, interaction between axons and Schwann cells, and angiogenesis [118].

2.1.2 Chitosan

Chitin is a biopolymer present in the shells of crustaceans and cuticle of and exoskeleton of arthropods [119]. Chitosan can be obtained from the chitin, by a process of partial deacetylation [120] commercially available by alkaline hydrolysis [121], and can be found in nature in some fungi [122]. Because of its characteristics, chitin, chitosan, and its complexes have already been explored for different medical and industrial applications, namely, for wound treatment, drug delivery systems, and space-filling implants. These biomaterials present positive features such as good biocompatibility and biodegradability; nontoxic character; low price; possibility of being modified chemically and enzymatically; antimicrobial properties; controlled release of components such as cytokines, antibiotics, and extracellular matrix components; promotion of cell adhesion; and maintenance of cell and tissue viabilities. These can also be shaped to create different forms, from films, sponges, or fibers to hydrogels and complex scaffolds [123, 124]. The described features turn these materials into adequate options for peripheral nerve reconstruction [125], with their potential to promote nerve regeneration demonstrated in vivo and in vitro [63]. One of the main disadvantages assigned to the use of chitosan matrices is its reduced mechanical strength when exposed to physiological conditions, failing to preserve its initial shape after implantation [126].

Chitosan conduits modified with different biodegradable polymers have been developed and evaluated.

Cheng et al. tested chitosan-poly(L-lysine) composite films, considering that the hydrophilic nature of chitosan appears to be essential to prevent the development of glial scars and promote nerve regeneration, observing enhanced cellular affinity and outcomes when compared to collagen films [127]. Similarly, the use of gelatin mixed with chitosan composite films displayed increased elasticity of the conduits and greater nerve cell affinity, besides promoting cell differentiation [128]. Wang et al. was able to improve nerve reparation along a large gap in the sciatic nerve of dogs using chitosan-polyglycolic acid (PGA) grafts, noting the reestablishment of nerve continuity and functional recovery [129].

Chitosan NGCs modified with inorganic components were also explored. In a study by Gärtner et al., chitosan tubes modified with apatite were used to improve their mechanical strength and avoid swelling. The application in the rat model of axonotmesis allowed the observation of neovascularization and macrophages phagocytizing cell debris, thus demonstrating functional Wallerian degeneration [130].

Itoh et al. studied the efficacy of chitosan tubes obtained from tendons of the *Macrocheira kaempferi* crab in the rat sciatic nerve submitted to neurotmesis. Some tubes also had laminin and laminin peptides adsorbed, to favor the adhesion of Schwann cells and the growth produced by the neurites. At weeks 2–4 post implantation, the tubes revealed inflammatory and macrophagic infiltration due to some fragmentation of the tube wall, with evidence of peripheral nerve regeneration after 6 weeks. In tubes enriched with laminin and laminin peptides, the regenerative process occurred over the internal wall, while in the other tube formulation, it was observed inside the lumen. Nociceptive function recovery was smaller than that observed with the use of isografts [131]. Wang et al. also confirmed that the use of chitosan laminin-peptide-treated tubes resulted in an increased number of regenerated axons, many of them adhering to the inner layer of the wall, that is, the one where these substances had been covalently bound with a nano-/microfiber mesh [125].

The use of chitosan in the form of nanocomposite, in association with gold, was also described. These nanoparticles improved the mechanical force of chitosan and stimulated the proliferation of neural cells and gene expression, thus resulting in better and faster functional recovery in a neurotmesis model, with more myelinated axons than the use of the isolated composite [132].

Wang created a nonwoven nano-/microfiber mesh tube comprising on an inner layer of a nano-/microfiber chitosan mesh and an outer layer of chitosan film. It was then used in the treatment of a rat sciatic nerve undergoing neurotmesis, comparing with simple chitosan nano-/microfiber mesh tubes and chitosan film tubes. The results showed that the chitosan nano-/microfiber mesh tubes displayed mechanical properties capable of preserving the tube space, guaranteeing a good scaffold for migration and cell adhesion, and facilitated the humoral flow that stimulates regeneration [123].

The importance of the acetylation of chitosan in promoting nerve regeneration was also identified by other authors. Freier et al. compared the compressive force of chitin gel tubes and chitosan tubes with different degrees of acetylation and concluded that the lesser the acetylation rate, the superior the mechanical strength, lower the degradation rate, and greater the adhesion and viability of the cells applied. The main factor in determining cell compatibility with chitosan was its charge, depending on the availability of amine groups. Since for lower degrees of acetylation there is an increase in charge density, it results in increased cell adhesion [121, 122]. In the works of Haastert-Talini et al. and Gonzalez-Perez et al., it was determined that the optimal degree of acetylation to stimulate nerve reparation is about 5%. Acetylation values around 2% cannot guarantee axonal regeneration, whereas acetylation around 20% degrades too early and has poor mechanical stability [133, 134].

The benefits of using chitosan may be improved by the modification of its properties but also by the concomitant use of other therapies such as growth factors or MSCs. The combined approaches aim to speed up the regenerative process and to decrease the secondary effects related to the degradation of chitosan. The chitosan polymer and its short chains do not cause an inflammatory response [135], but the fragments of its degradation can cause inflammation, leading to apoptosis of the regenerating cells and proliferation of fibrous tissue around the NGCs [119].

In the works of Patel et al., chitosan tubes enriched with laminin and GDNF were used [136]. GDNF is a trophic factor that promotes axonal regeneration, prevents atrophy of motor neurons, and relieves neuropathic pain [137]. Using this combination, nerves with a neurotmesis injury presented superior functional recovery to those submitted to unblended chitosan tubes. These results corroborate that, although they can promote nerve repair alone, isolated chitosan tubes have limited potential for regenerative promotion. Hsu et al. tested different tubes to promote nerve regeneration, comparing simple silicone tubes, laminin (LN)-modified chitosan scaffold in silicone conduit, and laminin (LN)-modified chitosan scaffold with bone marrow MSCs (BMSCs) combined with silicone conduit. The laminin (LN)-modified chitosan scaffold in silicone tubes was surrounded by macrophagic and eosinophilic hyperplasia granulation tissue after the experimental period, which was not observed in the presence of MSCs. This indicates that MSCs not only prevent the death of neurons and stimulate nerve regeneration but also reduce the inflammation and fibrotic development that may eventually be triggered by the long-term implantation of chitosan [138].

Lauto et al. tested the use of chitosan in PNI cases in a distinct perspective, developing an adhesive formula comprising chitosan, indocyanine green, acetic acid, and water. Applied in promoting rat tibial nerve regeneration, this alternative method promoted superior nerve repair, allowing connections between nerve ends stronger than those achieved with the use of fibrin glue. This chitosan adhesive presents several advantages when compared to traditional fibrin glue, namely, its insolubility in physiological fluids, its hydrophilicity, and presenting adhesiveness before laser activation [139].

The mechanical properties of the chitosan can be improved by an adjustment with a silane agent such as γ-glycidoxypropyltrimethoxysilane (GPTMS), improving its mechanical strength by promoting the wettability of chitosan surfaces. Some works have confirmed that integrating silicates into the chitosan membrane honed their cytocompatibility, making the combinations good candidates to be applied clinically [140–143]. Following these works, Amado et al. applied porous chitosan GPTMS membranes with about 110 μm pores and 90% of porosity in rat sciatic nerve injuries to study its effect on nerve regeneration [144]. The results showed that using porous hybrid chitosan membranes promoted a significantly better nerve fiber regeneration than solid membranes. The porous membranes, with a greater surface-to-volume ratio, showed the capacity to maintain mechanical strength [145] and the ability to adapt to different shapes. Its use allows an adequate revascularization of the regenerating tissue, reestablishment of metabolic communication with the surrounding microenvironment, and maintenance of nutrient and oxygen exchanges at adequate levels [146]. These conditions promote the proliferation of

Schwann cells, neurite extension, and remyelination, leading to an increased number of axons and nerve fibers and even increased thickness of myelin sheath [144].

Simões et al. also compared the use of solid and porous membranes in sciatic nerve axonotmesis and neurotmesis models, having observed a significant infiltration of multinucleated giant cells and some mast cells into the porous membrane and the development of an inflammatory reaction capsule with the solid membrane. These differences in the established inflammatory reactions may therefore justify the improved regeneration observed with the use of the porous membrane. Since the membranes with pores present a bigger surface-to-volume ratio, a higher contact with the immune system of the host can justify the greater infiltration of cells [147]. Simões et al. further compared the use of lacquered-poly(lactide-co-glycolic) acid test tubes with acetic acid and glycolic acid in a ratio of 90:10 (PLGA 90:10) with the use of chitosan porous membranes in the neurotmesis model through different surgical methods. The results revealed that although nerve regeneration occurred in all groups of animals, those with tubulization with chitosan presented better nerve regeneration and functional recovery than those receiving PLGA tubes [63]. A similar study was performed by Shirosaki et al., and the results also revealed that, although nerve regeneration was achieved in all experimental groups, chitosan porous hybrid tubulization was the treatment that promoted better nerve regeneration and functional recovery [141]. The ability of the porous chitosan GPTMS to promote nerve regeneration is probably related to its ability to promote the expression of genes related to myelin and the ions of silica that stimulate the expression of different glycoproteins [148]. This allows the nerve fibers to regenerate along the chitosan structure, establishing an extensive perineural connective architecture that ensures axonal fasciculation [63].

In June 2014, a commercial product was launched consisting of a chitosan-based nerve conduit with the name Reaxon® Nerve Guide, manufactured by Medovent GmbH (Mainz, Germany) and following the international standard DIN EN ISO 13485 [119]. The Reaxon® is flexible and resistant to collapse, and transparent, which facilitates the insertion of the nerve ends and the application of the anchoring sutures. The electrostatic interaction of the surface of Reaxon® Nerve Guide (positively charged) and the molecules or cells used in nerve repair (negatively charged) promotes the regenerative phenomena [149]. Fornasari et al. conducted a trial study on the mouse model using Reaxon® Nerve Guides, comparing the use of the commercial tube alone with a combination with muscular tissue (for the production of neuregulin 1, a stimulant of activity and survival of Schwann cells) and autografts. Both single tubes and tubes associated with skeletal muscle tissue positively promoted nerve regeneration and return to nerve function [150].

2.1.3 Synthetic nerve conduits

Polymers of synthetic origin have been applied in recent decades as a material for surgical sutures with relative success, and many of them have already been approved for clinical application. These materials present several advantages when used as scaffolds and neural tube guides. First, they can be adapted and produced in a wide variety of mechanical properties and degradation rates. Its well-described characteristics indicate a relatively low risk of immune reactions. Finally, the synthetic polymers can be combined to create new unique mechanical properties. Nevertheless, the biocompatibility of some of these materials may be reduced due to the difficulty of cells to adhere and survive.

Since non-biodegradable tube guides have the disadvantage of requiring a second surgery to remove the implant, research has focused on the development of biodegradable synthetic materials with an acceptable degradation time. The products resulting from degradation phenomena must not have toxic effects or trigger foreign body reactions. In addition, the biodegradable synthetic materials can be adapted towards the requirements necessary for their purpose, namely, serving as a support for the cellular systems used [151]. Examples of biodegradable synthetic materials are herein described:

2.1.4 Poly(lactic-co-glycolic acid)

Poly(lactic-co-glycolic acid), a copolymer resulting from the reaction between the biodegradable poly(glycolic acid) (PGA) and poly(lactic acid) (PLA), is one biomaterial presenting appropriate biocompatibility and biodegradability.

The isolated PGA is a rigid, thermostatic, highly crystalline polyester with high tensile modulus and high melting point but with low solubility in organic solvents. Its degradation leads to the production of glycolic acid, whose detrimental effects on growing cells are limited. Because of its hydrophilic nature, PGA has been used in the past to produce the first fully synthetic absorbable sutures [101]. A crimped PGA tube (Neurotube® Synovis Micro Companies Alliance, Birmingham, AL, USA) was approved as the first synthetic, highly porous, and bioresorbable NGCs approved by FDA in 1999 and was used for the repair of peripheral nerve injuries [152]. More recently, the use of BMSCs and Schwann-like cells (that had differentiated from BMSCs) in combination with Neurotube® in autografted rat facial nerves after neurotmesis was reported. At 6 weeks after surgery and application of the therapeutic combinations, it was found that facial nerve regeneration was improved by the cell therapy associated with PGA tubes [153]. However, PGA may also present some drawbacks. After implantation, ester bonds of the polymer may undergo hydrolysis, leading to degradation and production of derived metabolic products, triggering pH changes in the implantation site after organic absorption [101]. To improve the characteristics, PGA copolymers with PLA were developed, resulting in a more hydrophilic material.

PLA can be produced based on lactic acid obtained from natural products such as wheat, corn, or sugar beet, exhibiting good biocompatibility [154]. The speed of degradation of the scaffolds can be modified by varying the proportion of the different polymers. Lactic acid is more hydrophobic because of an extra methyl group, which not only limits water uptake by about 2% but also decreases hydrolysis rate compared to PGA [101], despite PGA being less soluble in organic solvents than PLA [155]. This biomaterial has been used as NGC in some studies. One study reports the application of PLA NGCs subjected to microabrasion in injured peripheral nerves of rat, promoting the regeneration of the nervous gap 8 weeks after the surgical intervention [156]. In a different study, a PLA nerve conduit obtained through a process of immersion precipitation was used to connect a 20-mm-long lesion in the sciatic nerve of the rabbit. These conduits sustained macropores in their external layer and micropores in their internal layer, allowing a better outflow rate than the inflow rate. This treatment resulted in up to 80% functional recovery after 18 months [157]. In another study, the authors compared the use of nerve conduits comprising PLA nonwoven fabric, silicone tubes filled with type I collagen gel, and autologous nerves in the regeneration of the buccal branch of the facial nerve presenting a 7 mm lesion. At 13 weeks after surgery, myelinization degree and axonal diameter were higher in the PLA tube-treated groups [158]. Still in another study, a microporous micro-patterned PLA obtained by photolithography was tested in the regeneration of a rat sciatic nerve with a 15 mm defect, with observation of good regeneration capacity and functional recovery, particularly when used with neural stem cells on the micro-patterned surfaces [159].

The copolymer of PLA and PGA (PLGA) presents increased hydration and degradation rates than the individual homopolymers [160] and has been described in multiple studies to assess for its ability to promote nerve regeneration [61]. Its most relevant features are its good biodegradability and biocompatibility and possible tuning of degradation time [161]. Its effectiveness is potentiated when combined with growth factors [162] and cell therapies [163, 164] or with the inclusion of a 3D support structure within the conduit [161]. Although these conduits show significantly better results than other biomaterials, they are not easily adaptable for different gap lengths nor for the release of different drugs. There are several drug delivery mechanisms described, such as microspheres, coatings, cross-linked polymers, or lumen filling with different solutions, but there is still little flexibility in the choice of active compounds and their concentrations in different PNI [165].

Over the years, PLGA has been one of the most frequently used biodegradable polymers for biomedical studies. Its degradation leads to the production of glycolic acid, and even if the effect of this product on the cells is reduced, PLGA degradation products are more acidic than other products such as collagen, which may eventually trigger changes in the underlying tissues [154]. Mechanically, its degradation characteristics can be controlled by changes in its molecular weight, copolymer ratio, and crystallinity, allowing for degradation periods varying from months to years, based on the proportion between the two polymers [166].

2.1.5 Poly(D,L-lactide-co-ε-caprolactone)

Poly-ε-caprolactone is an aliphatic, bioabsorbable, and biocompatible polyester commonly used in pharmaceuticals for wound treatment [167]. Its production is achieved by chemical synthesis from crude oil. Since PCL degrades by hydrolyzing its ester linkages under physiological conditions, it has gained prominence among implantable biomaterials. Poly(D,L-lactide-co-ε-caprolactone) (PCL) is a copolymer between the caprolactone and lactic acid monomers, and 80/20 copolymer nerve conduits can be produced by ink-jet systems [168]. Its degradation rate is slower than PLGA (about 16 months). In addition, the PCL degradation products are less acidic than those of PLGA, with less damage to the surrounding tissues. Finally, the PCL is transparent, making it easier to position the nerve stumps. However, its poor flexibility may hamper the microsurgical technique during implantation [164].

One study demonstrated that cells with genetic modifications to release NGF could adhere, survive, and release NGF for extended periods (>8 weeks) when cultured onto 80/20 PLA-PCL scaffolds, while 25/75 and 40/60 PLA-PCL copolymers were deemed unable to sustain cellular adhesion and survival [169]. Other studies demonstrated the in vivo biocompatibility of PCL membranes, tube guides, and nerve cells, facilitating cell adhesion, differentiation, and growth [144, 170].

Neurolac™ (commercially available PCL conduit) application in vivo results in conflicting reports. While some studies have attest the efficacy of PCL to promote both morphological recoveries and functional improvements in neurotmesis and axonotmesis lesions of rat sciatic nerves [170, 171], others report no beneficial effects [172]. Luís et al. compared the effectiveness of PLGA 90/10 and PCL NGCs in helping nerve regeneration along the 10 mm gap of the rat sciatic nerve, further comparing this material with conventional approaches of end-to-end neurorrhaphy and autologous graft. Both types of biomaterials promoted functional improvements and were considered as good options for tubular NGCs, and their degradation characteristics did not seem to have an impact over the level of nerve regeneration. After the 20-week study period, PGLA presented accelerated biodegradation when compared to PCL [170]. The efficacy of PCL membranes (Vivosorb™) in the promotion of nerve regeneration after neurotmesis was tested in combination with MSCs from the Wharton's jelly (WJMSCs), demonstrating the differentiation of the MSCs into neuroglia-like cells, expressing specific phenotypical markers. In vivo tests performed over 20 weeks resulted in functional recovery and significant morphometric improvements [164].

2.1.6 Polyvinyl alcohol

Polyvinyl alcohol (PVA) is a nondegradable and water-soluble polymer whose potentialities to be used as NGC have recently been explored [173–175]. Currently there is a non-absorbable PVA hydrogel (SaluBridge, SaluTunnel, SaluMedica LCC, Atlanta, GA, USA). Its 3D nanofibrillation structure confers exceptional biocompatibility, water intake capacity, elasticity, mobility and saturability, and high resistance to mechanical deformation [176]. In one study, a tubular PVA conduit was tested for its effects over axonal growth using rat dorsal root ganglia, considering its wall thickness, its level of porosity, and the Schwann cell seeding density. It was identified that lower porosity and higher wall thickness delayed the regeneration of the axons, with the best results observed with 75% porosity, associated with Schwann cell-seeded conduits [177].

More recent studies address the combination of PVA with other materials. Ribeiro et al. studied the effect of PVA loaded with electrically conductive materials (polypyrrole and carbon nanotubes) on axonotmesis injuries. The combination of PVA and carbon nanotubes displayed improved biocompatibility, electrical conductivity, and better histomorphometric results [178]. After neurotmesis injury, the association of MSCs with the PVA, carbon nanotubes promoted better nerve fiber regeneration, suggesting a positive synergistic effect [179].

3. Cellular systems

Historically, neural-derived cellular systems were the first to be proposed for neural tissue regeneration (as the N1E-115) and are briefly addressed herein. Later, MSCs isolated form a variety of niches that have been proposed for the purpose, and some populations are gaining prominence due to technical and ethical minutiae, such as perinatal, dental, and olfactory mucosa-derived MSCs (**Table 2**).

MSC	Classification	Advantages and Mechanism of Action
N1E-115	Neuroblastoma cell line	• Increase the local concentration of neurotrophic factors.
Fetal-derived Mesenchymal Stem Cell	Multipotent stem cells	• Augment the blood perfusion; • Enhance intraneural vascularity; • Differentiate into Schwann-like cells; • Produce and release varied neurotrophic factors; • Collection usually does not require surgical intervention; • Less immunoreactivity.
Dental Pulp Mesenchymal Stem Cells	Multipotent stem cell	• Promote axonal growth and guidance; • Promote and guides myelinization; • Stronger harvesting and proliferation potential; • Great clonogenic potential.
Olfactory Mucosa Mesenchymal Stem Cells	Multipotent stem cell	• Promote neural differentiation; • Produce neurotrophic factors; • Promote maturation of glial cells; • Activate myelination *in vitro;* • Easy collection and isolation.

Table 2.
Summary of characteristics of the cellular systems used by our research group in cell-based therapies for PNI research.

3.1 N1E-115 cells

Neurotrophic factors may stimulate several important components of neural regeneration process, involving the survival and regrowth of sensory and motor nerve fibers. Thus, in vivo Schwann cell differentiation and axon remyelination [180] may vary depending on the method of releasing these factors. The delivery devices must be highly complex to allow controlled release. In this context, N1E-115, a cell line obtained from mouse neuroblastoma C-1300 [181] and able to follow a neurodifferentiation when exposed to dimethylsulfoxide [182], adenosine 3′;5′-cyclic monophosphate [183] or serum removal started to be studied.

These cells were already used in both axonotmesis and neurotmesis lesions because of its capacity to produce and deliver different neurotrophic factors capable to promote axonal regeneration [184]. The advantage in using N1E-115 cells to increase the local concentration of neurotrophic factors is thought to be related to the fact that the concentration of these factors is similar to those observed in endogenous cell production and they are released directly in the proximity of the region under regeneration. The measurement of $[Ca^{2+}]_i$ allowed to establish 48h under differentiation as the appropriated period, presenting N1E-115 cells in this moment characteristics of neurons without entering the process of cell death associated with $[Ca^{2+}]$ modifications [184, 185].

Different studies were performed to infer on the pro-regenerative capacity of the N1E-115 cell line in the peripheral nerve injury, associating these cells with biomaterials such as collagen [104, 111], hybrid chitosan [144], and PLGA 90/10 [186]. Despite all the expected advantages of using biomaterials in association with these cells, the results obtained did not show a special efficacy of N1E-115 cells in promoting nerve regeneration regardless of the type of lesion [144]. Only slight motor improvements were observed with the combination of collagen and N1E-115 in axonotmesis lesions, while no improvements were noted in neurotmesis lesions previously submitted to end-to-end suture. No functional improvements and poor morphometric regeneration was obtained from the use with PLGA [186]. It was hypothesized that the physical presence of N1E-115 cells at nerve scaffolds may have generated a consumption of local blood supplied nutrients and oxygen, arresting the positive effect of local neurotrophic factor release.

3.2 Perinatal mesenchymal stem cells

Perinatal tissues represent the most primitive MSC niches after the embryonic stage and those that have suffered the least genetic alterations because of environmental exposure, aging, or occurrence of pathological changes [187]. Among these tissues, MSCs can be obtained from different sites, namely, umbilical cord blood and stroma (Wharton's jelly), amniotic fluid, and membrane (**Figure 4a**).

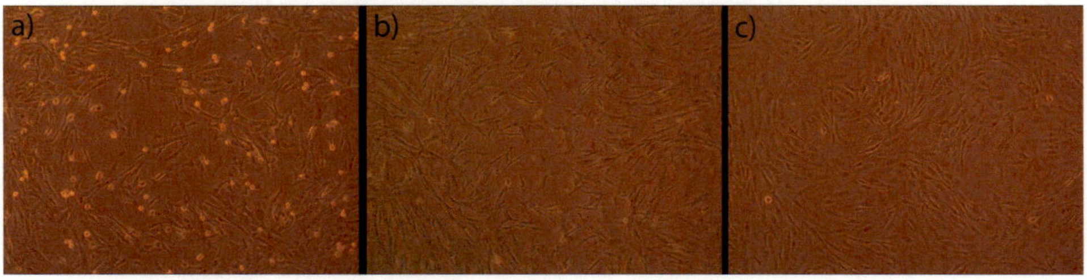

Figure 4.
(a) Equine UC-MSCs in culture (P1). (b) Human dental pulp MSCs in culture (P2). (c) Rat olfactory mucosa MSCs in culture (P4). Magnification: 100×.

Since perinatal tissues are traditionally discarded after birth, MSCs can be isolated through noninvasive procedures. Once isolated, it is easy to establish cultures with these cells and promote their neural differentiation [188, 189]. The list of advantages associated with the use of MSCs with perinatal origin includes the fact that they allow an autologous cell source, are easily processed and cryopreserved, and present low immunogenicity. Besides that, they have a low tumorigenic potential when compared to other types of MSCs [190] and have excellent cell growth capacities. The quality of these cells can vary between patients, depending on the specific characteristics of the tissues of each donor, the transport time, the conditions to which the cells were subjected during the same, and the processing and cryopreservation techniques applied [191].

The umbilical cord stroma (Wharton's jelly) is a singular primitive proteoglycan connective tissue that protects the blood vessels of the umbilical cord and the cells within [192]. The amount of cells that can be isolated from the Wharton's jelly (WJMSCs) is comparatively superior than those that can be isolated from other niches. These cells lack the expression of hematopoietic markers [99, 193], express low levels of histocompatibility complex (MHC) class I, are negative to MHC II, are also easily expanded in culture and plastic adherent, exhibit a normal fibroblastic-like shape [190], and have excellent population doubling times [194]. The in vitro differentiation capacity of these cells is also ample towards several mesodermal cell types such as osteocytes, chondrocytes, adipocytes, skeletal myocytes, cardiomyocytes, hepatocytes, insulin-producing cells, and, of particular importance, neuron-like cells which differentiate when exposed to a neurogenic culture medium for a period of 96 h [190]. WJMSCs have the capacity not only to differentiate into Schwann-like cells but also to produce and release varied neurotrophic factors such as BDNF, NGF, and neurotrophin-3, stimulating axonal growth in vitro [195]. In addition, transformed MSCs still present viability during 4 months after transplantation without any need to institute immune suppression [188].

WJMSCs have already been used to promote the regeneration of different tissues in combination with biomaterials with relative success. Using WJMSCs associated with a PVA membrane to treat chronic cutaneous lesions showed good levels of skin regeneration and reduction in number and extension of ulcers [196]; the use of WJMSCs and their conditioned medium (CM) in association with gelatin matrix scaffolds (commercially available haemostatic sealant, Floseal®) in promoting regeneration of myectomy lesions revealed good functional and histological improvements, although some long-term negative effects were detected and not observed in the treatment with CM. The CM obtained from the culture of WJMSCs can be, therefore, a suitable alternative to the in vivo application of these cells [197].

Regarding the efficacy of WJMSCs in peripheral nerve regeneration after injury, several studies have already been performed. The addition of WJMSCs to NGCs seems to bring advantages related to the production and secretion of neurotrophic and angiogenic factors that improve the local regenerative environment. Animals submitted to neurotmesis present greater functional and sensory improvements when treated with WJMSCS in combination with biodegradable NGCs than when treated with single NGCs [99]. The combined use of WJMSCs with PVA guide tubes loaded with electrically conductive materials (carbon nanotubes and polypyrrole) was able to prevent the occurrence of neurogenic muscular atrophy and reestablish the neuromuscular junction, with the use of MSCs with PVA loaded with carbon nanotubes being effective in inducing a bigger amount of regenerated fibers and thicker myelin sheets. Similarly, the use of PCL and MSCs in neurotmesis lesions immediately submitted to end-to-end sutures also seemed to bring special advantages in terms of motor function recovery, probably because of local secretion of growth factors and cytokines [193].

Still within the use of MSCs from perinatal tissues in peripheral nerve regeneration, treatment of the rat sciatic nerve after neurotmesis with Floseal® as cell vehicle for WJMSCs mediated the Wallerian degeneration stage, improving the subsequent regeneration and the morphology of the nerve fibers. It promoted a lesser extent of fibrosis in the acute phase of the lesion, besides a chronic phase where a greater thickness of the myelin sheets and a larger number of regenerated fibers have been observed. Positive functional and morphological effects in both acute and chronic phases revealed a positive synergistic effect [198].

3.3 Dental pulp mesenchymal stem cells

The dental pulp is the most internal layer of the tooth and is composed of loose connective tissue that includes blood vessels, nerves, and mesenchymal tissue, having an important function in the primary and secondary development of teeth and in resolving pathological processes such as caries [199]. The formation of odontoblasts and the production of dentin in response to severe lesions in the teeth were precisely the first suggestive signs of the presence of MSCs in the dental pulp. Dental pulp mesenchymal stem cells (DPSCs) were isolated for the first time at the beginning of the last decade from a third molar and demonstrated to be able to differentiate into odontoblast-like cells [200]. Over time DPSCs have been isolated from exfoliated deciduous teeth, human permanent and primary teeth, supernumerary teeth [199], and teeth of various nonhuman species [201]. They exhibit all the characteristics of MSCs that make them appropriate options for clinical application, being capable of following multi-lineage differentiation, (including neural differentiation [202]) when under suitable culture conditions; presenting self-renewal capacity [203]; expressing MSC phenotypic markers [204], stemness-related markers, cytoskeleton-related markers [205]; and, as expected, not expressing hematopoietic markers (**Figure 4b**) [203]. Specifically, DPSCs express neural markers [206, 207]; produce neurotrophic factors; stimulate the differentiation, growth, and orientation of growing axons; and differentiate into active and functional neurons [208, 209]. Compared to other types of MSCs, DPSCs have higher clonogenic capacity, high proliferation, and a larger stem/progenitor cell population. DPSC source tissues are, like perinatal tissues, readily collectible without additional harm to the donor or invasive surgical procedures [210], and isolated cells can be used autologously as long as their characteristics are maintained through good isolation and cryopreservation protocols.

DPSCs secrete different trophic factors that stimulate nerve regeneration and showed ability to chemo-attract trigeminal ganglion axons [211], guiding myelin repair and stimulating dorsal root ganglion neurite outgrowth [212, 213]. Besides its efficacy to stimulate regeneration of other tissues [214], some work has been performed to attest the ability of DPSCs to stimulate peripheral nerve regeneration after PNI. The use of silicone tubes filled with DPSCs embedded in collagen gel proved to be effective in promoting regeneration of the rat facial nerve after injury [215]. The same authors further assessed degradable PLGA tubes filled with DPSCs embedded in collagen gel, which were able to stimulate regeneration and functional recovery of the rat sciatic nerve after neurotmesis [216]. The use of collagen devices filled with Schwann-like cells induced from DPSCs also resulted in nerve repair and regeneration in sciatic nerves of rats with 15 mm gap [217]. Martens et al. proved not only the ability of DPSCs to differentiate into Schwann cells with increased glial marker expression and secretion of neurotrophic factors but also the ability of these differentiated cells to promote axonal outgrowth and myelination in 2D or 3D culture conditions in an in vitro model [212]. In addition, the synergistic use of DPSCs and Schwann cells with nerve conduits in solving 15 mm gap lesions in the rat sciatic nerve was demonstrated to be more effective in restoring nerve conduction velocity than the use of DPSCs and nervous conduits alone [218]. Knowing the importance of oligodendrocyte lineage transcription factor 2 in the oligodendrogenic pathway, Askari et al. were capable to induce the differentiation of DPSCs into oligodendrocytes by transfection of a tetracycline (Tet)-inducible system expressing oligodendrocyte lineage transcription factor 2 gene. These differentiated cells were then used in the treatment of a local demyelinating lesion of the mouse sciatic nerve by lysolecithin, with observation of repair and regeneration of the injured nerve [209]. The comparative use of DPSCs and neuronal cells originating from the differentiation of DPSCs in the treatment of a 5 mm lesion in the rat sciatic nerve proved that both cell types promoted functional and muscle contraction improvements, associated with the identification of specific markers for angiogenesis, even though no specific differences between the two cell types in promoting nerve regeneration were identified [219]. Furthermore, in a model of diabetic polyneuropathy, DPSC transplantation promoted the secretion of several cytokines that were capable of modulating the M1/M2 macrophage proportions and promoting anti-inflammatory effects, besides increasing the velocity of nerve conduction and local nerve blood flow [220].

In summary, DPSCs have the remarkable capacity to not only produce and release neurotrophic factors with protective immune modulative functions at the site of nerve damage but also to differentiate into oligodendrocyte-like and Schwann-like cells.

3.4 Olfactory mucosa mesenchymal stem cells

In the *lamina propria* of mammal olfactory mucosa, a different MSC population can be found: the olfactory mucosa mesenchymal stem cells (OM-MSCs). This lineage has also been called ectomesenchymal stem cells because of their ectodermal origin and the fact that they express neural cell-related genes [221]. The OM-MSCs have been identified and studied in different extents in diverse species such as humans [221], mouse [222], rabbit [223], dog [224], sheep, horse, macaque, and lemur [225], although they were initially found and identified at the rat olfactory mucosa [226]. Some studies were carried out and allowed an initial characterization of these cells, namely, the identification of their MSCs characteristics when in culture (plastic adhesion and capacity to form fibroblastic-like low density colonies) and the expression of classic MSC markers and of those related to differentiations (**Figure 4c**) [221]. In fact, OM-MSCs not only are capable of performing classical tri-differentiation but also have the ability to myogenic and neurogenic differentiation [227]. Additionally, its CM can promote the proliferation of ensheathing cells and oligodendrocyte precursor cells and also activate myelination in vitro [228]. OM-MSCs present features that put them in the list of cells to be used in regenerative medicine, namely, its high versatility, wide distribution in nasal cavity with easy access, few ethical issues, good location for both *antemortem* and *postmortem* collection (particularly in larger donors), neural crest origin, and little tendency for development of chromosomal or tumorigenic alterations [229, 230]. Finally, OM-MSCs maintain self-renewal ability in culture for long periods of time by conserving telomeric activity and inhibiting apoptotic activity, without the age seeming to affect this characteristic [231].

The study of OM-MSCs secretome led to the identification of several molecules with the capacity to promote effects on neural differentiation and production and maturation of glial cells [81]. From a clinical application point of view, besides the studies carried out to test its potential in the control of autoimmune diseases [232, 233] and in the regeneration of myocardial tissue after infarct [234], OM-MSCs have already shown regenerative efficacy when used as therapy in degenerative diseases of the CNS [235], hippocampal lesions [236, 237], lesions associated with hearing loss [238–240], and in cases of spinal cord trauma [241, 242]. Regarding its effectiveness in promoting peripheral nerve regeneration after PNI, the studies and data obtained are still reduced to allow definitive conclusions. Roche et al. carried out a work in which they studied the efficacy of OM-MSCs delivered in an NGC comprising of a biphasic laminin and collagen-functionalized hyaluronic acid, testing its efficacy on the regeneration of a rat sciatic nerve with a 10 mm gap, with and without NGF supplementation. It was identified that animals treated with OM-MSCs and implantation of NGCs showed clinical and electrophysiological improvements and a nociceptive recovery superior to those identified in the animals that only received NGCs [243].

4. Microsurgical procedures

As in most biomedical works, mouse and rat are the most frequently used models in the studies of peripheral nerve regeneration. Our research group works mainly with the rat model, Sasco Sprague-Dawley breed. The anatomy of the rat is well characterized, presenting many similarities with men's peripheral nerves. Being a small model, the rat still presents nerves with significant dimensions, facilitating the performance of the microsurgical interventions and allowing standardization and comparison of the functional tests performed. In terms of dimensions and density of connective tissue, there are differences in comparison to human nerves, and the biggest disadvantage of using small rodents is their high intrinsic neural regeneration capacity, which can sometimes make it difficult to determine the translational value of the therapeutic methods applied [244, 245]. Regarding the nerve model, most studies explore the sciatic nerve and its terminal branches, particularly because of the dimensions of this nerve [246] and the high number of functional and behavioral tests available, mostly in the rat model [247]. Obviously, the high number of data accessible in the literature allows an effective comparison with the results observed in previous work. The most common types of experimental lesion paradigms include the induction of crush injuries that lead to axonal functional interruption with maintenance of connective sheaths (axonotmesis), disruption of the nerve trunk through a complete transection, or removal of a segment with creation of a gap with specific dimensions (neurotmesis) [248].

In our works, animals are operated under anesthesia and with adequate analgesia. With the animal in lateral decubitus, the trichotomy and asepsis of the area to intervene is performed, and the access to the sciatic nerve is made through a skin incision that extends from the greater trochanter to the distal mid-half of the hind limb and a dissection of the gluteal muscles. Once the sciatic nerve and its main branches are exposed with the aid of soft tissue retractors, the pretended lesion can be induced with a straight microsurgical scissors for neurotmesis lesions or crushing clamps for axonotmesis lesions. The lesion should be induced as distally as possible, preferably directly above the terminal nerve ramification. In neurotmesis lesions, both nerve ends are introduced about 3 mm inside the NGCs with or without associated cells, with the application of 7/0 monofilament nylon epineural sutures to keep nerve tops aligned, secure, and with a gap of desired dimensions. For neurotmesis lesions where there is no intention to maintain a gap, the nerve can be subjected to an end-to-end suture using 7/0 monofilament nylon, with or without posterior application of an NGC. For axonotmesis lesions, the biomaterial can be placed wrapping the crushing site and sutured. The cellular systems can be combined to the biomaterial conduit before (cultured and expanded on the biomaterial surface), during (infiltrated into the conduit in suspension or in a soft biomaterial vehicle, at the time of implantation), or after reconstruction (through direct injection within the nerve gap). Once this phase is concluded, the gluteal muscles can be sutured, isolated, or simultaneously with the skin, applying a simple-interrupted suture with a non-absorbable material. The contralateral limb is not intervened and used as a control. Animals submitted to surgery should be daily monitored to accompany the healing process and the recovery of nerve function [3].

5. Functional evaluation

In the studies involving sciatic nerve regeneration, the animal is followed postoperatively during 12 weeks for axonotmesis lesions [111] and 20 weeks for neurotmesis lesions [104], assuming that after this period functional and morphologic recovery is complete and can be determined. To determine the level of nerve regeneration, both morphological and functional results are considered in both types of lesions, although the correlation between the two types of data is not always strong [249]. The more classic and modern methods for determining nerve recovery, such as retrograde labeling [250] histomorphometry and histology [251], electrophysiological assessment [252], and in vivo imaging [253], rarely succeed in adequately revealing the reestablishment of motor and sensory functions, being more effective in the study of the regenerative process from the physiologic/structural point of view than in the assessment of effective functional recovery [254]. Thus, PNI research studies need to combine both functional and morphological assessment. Our works generally involves conducting a behavioral analysis, combined with histology, histomorphometry, and kinematic analysis (**Figure 5**).

5.1 Behavioral and functional analysis

Regarding motor function of the sciatic nerve, the test used to determine its recovery is the evaluation of SFI through the use of a walking track. First described in 1982 [255], the SFI is a quantitative and noninvasive method that allows to determine the recovery of the hind limb using methods of observation and recording of the rat's footprints, considering for this the spatial relation between the toes, the foot, and the hind limb as a whole [256]. Although it is a very popular test among PNI researchers, its validity is still questioned [257]. The major limitation

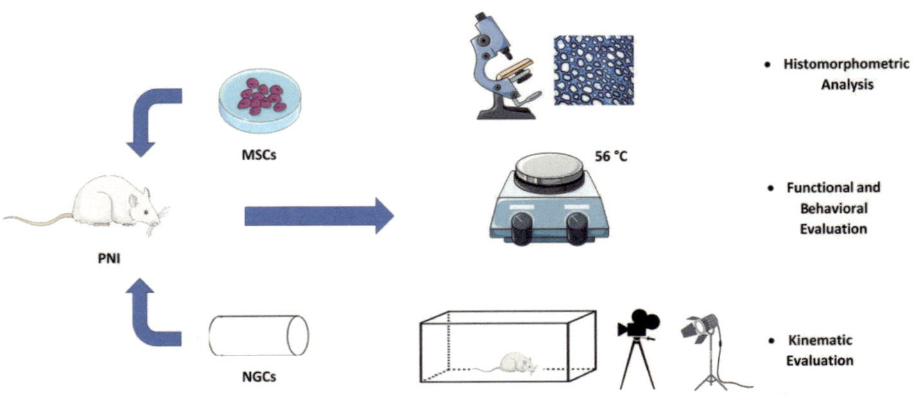

Figure 5.
Schematic representation of evaluation components used in works of our research group.

of the method is that animals frequently develop contractile flexions and autotomy, which consequently leads to defective and blurred paw records because of changes in limb placement or tail dragging during the footprint record, making it difficult to analyze [258]. To perform the test, the animals are confined within a 42-cm-long and 8.2-cm-wide walkway that ends in a dark shelter without exit. A white paper is placed on the floor of the walking corridor for registration. The hind paws of the rats are gently pressed onto the finger paint-soaked sponge to be impregnated with ink, and the animals are then placed at the beginning of the walkway to advance along the corridor and leave their hind paw records over the paper. Animals are always trained to walk in the corridor prior to surgery to stablish an individual baseline. Walking tracks are recorded preoperatively (week 0), after surgery at weeks 1 and 2, and from there every 2 weeks until week 12 or 20. In each record it is possible to make several measurements: print length (PL), distance from the heel to the third toe; toe spread (TS), distance from the first to the fifth toe; and intermediate toe spread (ITS), distance from the second to the fourth toe. Associated with the SFI, SSI is also determined, in which only the TS and ITS parameters are considered. SSI and SFI measurements are made on both the control and injured limbs. The average of three measurements are used in the following formulas: Toe spread factor (TSF) = (ETS – NTS)/NTS; Intermediate toe spread factor (ITSF) = (EITS – NITS)/NITS; Print length factor (PLF) = (EPL – NPL)/NPL, with E and N representing the injured and non-injured limbs, respectively. Finally, the SFI is calculated using the formula of Bian et al. [259]: SFI = −38.3 (EPL – NPL)/NPL + 109.5 (ETS – NTS)/NTS + 13.3 (EIT – NIT)/NIT – 8.8 = (−38.3 × PLF) + (109.5 × TSF) + (13.3 × ITSF) – 8.8. Alternatively, or complementarily, SSI is a fast index that is calculated without considering the PL value, using the equation: SSI = [(108.44 × TSF) + (31.85 × ITSF)] − 5.49. For both cases, a value of 0 is normal, and the closer the value is to −100, the worse the functional recovery. In situations where footprints cannot be measured, the value of −100 is automatically assigned. The footprints of each animal must be observed and analyzed by a single operator.

The method to test the motor performance is the EPT test [260], which consists in determining the force, measured in grams, that the animal is capable to exert with the injured and healthy limbs over a digital scale. This is an important test because for its correct accomplishment the animal needs to activate the muscles of the plantar flexor group (gastrocnemius and soleus), and the obtained values are correlated with those observed in the SFI and SSI [257]. To perform this test, the animal's body is wrapped in a surgical towel, leaving the hind limbs exposed. The animal must be supported by the thorax as it is lowered towards the digital balance. As hind limbs approach the balance, the EPT is elicited by the anticipation of the contact of the distal metatarsus with the balance, and the hind limbs are extended. The force, in grams, exerted over the balance is then registered. The method should be performed on both the affected and the healthy limb, being repeated three times to consider the average result. To determine the functional deficit percentage, normal limb (NEPT) and injured limb (EEPT) EPT values are then included in the following equation [261]: Percentage motor deficit = [(NEPT – EEPT) /NEPT] × 100. Animals are tested before surgery (week 0), week 1 and 2 after surgery, and from there every 2 weeks to week 12 or 20. EPT values are originally determined in grams of weight applied by each limb but are subsequently expressed as percentage deficit of the injured limb relatively to the weight applied by the healthy limb. The main limitations of the test relate to the operator's experience and comfort in handling animals. The operator also needs to have enough experience to recognize when the animal is applying as much force as possible with the limb to be tested. Since the operator is comfortable performing the test, it is highly reproducible [261].

Regarding the sensorial recovery of the sciatic nerve, the most used test is the WRL, also used in works of our research group. The WRL test, with the aim of establishing the maintenance or recovery of the nociceptive function, can be performed using a mechanical stimulation and electrical stimulation, by puncturing with a needle or, more commonly, with a heating plate [262]. Using a hot plate is not only the most common but also the most practical method. The nociceptive stimulation is applied on the hindpaw's plantar surface, determining the withdrawal reflex, that is, the time, in seconds, that the animal takes to retract the paw. Animals with sensory integrity retract the limbs more quickly from the nociceptive stimulus source [263]. To perform the test, the animal is covered with a surgical towel, and the limb to be tested is placed over the hotplate at 56°C, the time it takes to retract the limb being then recorded. In a healthy animal, the limb is retracted in around 4.3 s or less [264]. Limbs are tested three times, with a 2-min interval between each test to avoid sensitizations, and the result of three measurements is considered, on average, to get the final result. If the animal does not retract the limb within 12 s, it is removed from the heat stimulus to prevent tissue damage. The animals are tested before surgery (week 0), at week 1 and 2 after surgery, and from there every 2 weeks until week 12 or 20.

5.2 Kinematic analysis

The evaluation of locomotion quality is of utmost importance since this function integrates the sensory and motor systems and their constituents, including the nervous fibers of afferent and efferent nature, the sensory nerve terminations, the skeletal muscles, and the respective central integration centers. With the convenience of advanced image record devices, it is now possible to use digital technologies to more accurately evaluate gait analysis [265]. The kinematic evaluation is the set of analyses directed to the articular movements without considering the force that is being applied. Considering that branches of the sciatic nerve are responsible for the innervation of dorsiflexor and plantarflexor muscles, the set of kinematic evaluations used in this nerve, with video capture and later observation, include the determination of ankle kinematic, the measurement of gait stance duration, and evaluation of toe out angle during the gait [257]. The main disadvantage of kinematic evaluation is its technical complexity and the need for specific digital material.

In the studies conducted by our group (**Figure 6**), the kinematic evaluation of the ankle is performed considering the sagittal plane during the stance phase of walking after the induction of different injuries [104, 111]. Animals are encouraged to walk voluntarily throughout a corridor with two dark shelters at both ends to serve as a refuge, thus allowing the two-dimensional ankle motion analysis. The side walls of the corridors are transparent, and a high-speed video camera is positioned in an orthogonal position relatively to the corridor to record the ankle motion during the walk. Sagittal records are also considered, using a rate of 100 frames per second. The recorded images are scanned in a semiautomatic process resorting to marks placed at reference points over the rat hind limb and paw. By this procedure it is possible to get the trajectories of the leg and hindfoot segments, and the ankle joint angle is derived by using appropriate computation systems. The parameters for ankle kinematics proposed by Varejão et al. [266] are then applied to determine the sciatic functional recovery after injury and repair, so that therapeutic efficacies can be compared.

It is important, however, to realize that ankle kinematics should only be regarded as an indirect sign of muscle function. Animal locomotion requires the use of fine coordination of limbs, and quadruped animals can develop mobility strategies to compensate deficits in hind limbs. Through the plastic activation of integrative structures, the animal can develop patterns of adaptive movement that are observed

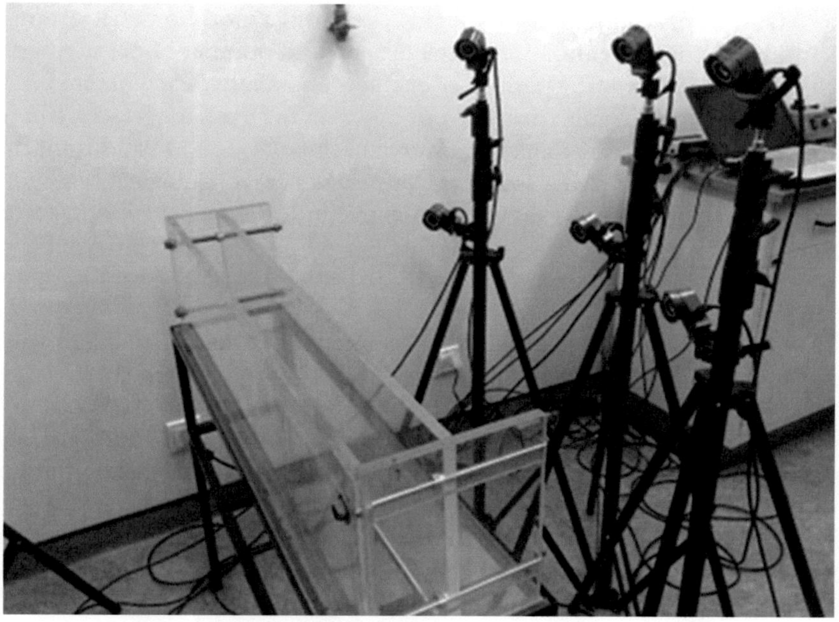

Figure 6.
Corridor and data capture chamber setup for kinematic evaluation in works of our research group.

even in the presence of severe denervation. In addition, a direct relationship between the results of simpler motor and sensory function tests and those got in the evaluation of the complex walking action is rarely observed [266, 267]. To achieve a precise assessment of functional recovery, walking analysis after PNI should evolve both the ankle kinematics analysis to a detailed description of the biomechanical and the mobility function of the hind limb, including a complete assessment of hip, knee, and ankle joints.

6. Morphological analysis

The morphological and histological evaluation of the injured nerve after the experimental period is a commonly used method to identify the size, organization, and number of regenerated nerve fibers and the thickness of the myelin sheath formed after PNI. Although morphological and histological evaluation was only descriptive in its earlier applications, it is now possible to perform morphometric and quantitative analysis of the histological sections to be studied, ideally in combination with other alternative methods of functional, electrophysiological, and molecular evaluation [251]. Quantitative analysis is important to identify both intact and regenerated axons, inflammation, and fibrotic reactions inside the nerve or in the form of perineural adhesions, besides the development of neuromas. The histomorphometric assessment also allows to identify the amount, type, and diameter of the cells that occupy a certain space within the nerve and the proportion of regenerated and healthy tissue [268]. When the efficacy of biomaterials is assessed, histological evaluation is essential to determine the level of material degradation, the development of granulomas and adherences, and the establishment of foreign body reactions [39].

The toluidine blue staining of semithin sections is the method more commonly applied for the histological characterization of the nerve after PNI. This technique allows the observation of the myelinated axons and to delimitate the myelin sheaths. Likewise, this method is adequate to perform a morphometric examination that leads to the determination of the density and number of nerve fibers, the cross-section dimensions, the perimeter of fibers and axons, the diameter of the fibers and axons, the different proportions between the axon diameters, fibers and myelin sheaths, and also the thickness of myelin sheaths [269]. In addition, this method also enables the evaluation of the ultrastructural changes caused by the regenerative phenomena in axons and in the myelin through transmission electron microscopy [270].

Regardless of the protocol considered, the histological and morphological evaluation of the nerve requires consolidated experience from the operator. It is necessary that the operator has a thorough knowledge about the anatomy of the nerve, about the histology of its segments, and about the differences between the same nerve sites in different animals. These knowledges are essential during the determination of the dimensions and number of myelinated fibers. The use of randomized protocols, biased measurements, and biased counting methodologies allows to prevent the occurrence of bias in the histological and morphometric evaluations. The morphological methods used to test axonal regeneration do not always allow to directly correlate the functional recovery and the level of axonal regeneration, and appropriate axonal regeneration and low functional outcomes are common occurrences. Moreover, because of the occurrence of protruding, separation, divergence, kinking, or straddling observed between the two portions of axons, histological evaluation can hinder the assessment of the nerve reparation. Finally, even with the high-resolution optical microscopy, myelinated fibers with a diameter infersior to 2 μm are hard to detect, potentially misjudging the counting [271].

7. Conclusions

PNI continue to bear enormous impact on the patient's quality of life, leading to significant functional deficits, disabilities, and substantial social and professional constraints. Significant advances in neural reparation and translational neurophysiology have been achieved through the refinement of microsurgery techniques, the comprehension of anatomy and topography of the nerve, and the understanding of pathophysiologic and molecular mechanisms related to PNI. Nerve reparation by epineural neurorrhaphy is still the preferred yet invasive approach in situations where tension-free alignment in a well-vascularized environment can be guaranteed. For larger gaps between the two nerve segments, this technique is not always adequate, and nerve grafting presents as the treatment of choice. In severe avulsion injuries, such as in the brachial plexus, nerve transfer techniques are also an option. The current most promising research lines in nerve regeneration are based on attempted strategies to accelerate reparation using sophisticated nerve conduits in combination with cell-based therapies. Several types of biomaterials with different physical presentations have been explored, demonstrating attractive pro-regenerative properties. This therapeutic potential is further boosted through its combination with cells, CM, and growth factors, indicating that combinatory therapies are the most promising strategy in regenerative medicine and PNI.

This chapter summarizes the principles of peripheral nerve injury and the observations gathered by our research group in this field over the years. This gathered knowledge results from the exploitation of diverse hypothesized therapeutic combination based on the use of biomaterials and cellular systems, achieving promising results. Nonetheless, there is still a long road ahead in this research area towards the achievement of optimal PNI recovery, and conclusions presented in currently available literature provide basis for further studies necessary for the consolidation of the proposed therapies.

Acknowledgements

This research was supported by Programa Operacional Regional do Norte (ON.2—O Novo Norte), QREN, FEDER with the project "iBone Therapies: Terapias inovadoras para a regeneração óssea," ref. NORTE-01-0247-FEDER-003262, and by the program COMPETE—Programa Operacional Factores de Competitividade, Projects PEst-OE/AGR/UI0211/2011 and PEst-C/EME/UI0285/2013 funding from FCT. This research was also supported by Programa Operacional Competitividade e Internacionalização (P2020), Fundos Europeus Estruturais e de Investimento (FEEI), and FCT with the project "BioMate—A novel bio-manufacturing system to produce bioactive scaffolds for tissue engineering" with reference PTDC/EMS-SIS/7032/2014 and by COMPETE 2020, from ANI—Projectos ID&T Empresas em Copromoção, Programas Operacionais POCI, by the project "insitu.Biomas—Reinvent biomanufacturing systems by using an usability approach for in situ clinic temporary implants fabrication" with the reference POCI-01-0247-FEDER-017771. Ana Rita Caseiro (SFRH/BD/101174/2014) and Rui Damásio Alvites (SFRH/BD/116118/2016) acknowledge FCT, for financial support.

Conflict of interest

The authors of this paper do not declare any conflict of interest regarding the content of the document.

Acronyms and abbreviations

AFMSCs	amniotic fluid mesenchymal stem cells
ALP	alkaline phosphatase
BDNF	brain-derived neurotrophic factor
BMSCs	bone marrow MSCs
CM	conditioned medium
DPSCs	dental pulp mesenchymal stem cells
EPT	extensor postural thrust
GDNF	glial cell-derived neurotrophic factor
GPTMS	glycidoxypropyltrimethoxysilane
ITS	intermediate toe spread
ITSF	intermediate toe spread factor
MHC	histocompatibility complex
MSC's	mesenchymal stem cells
NGCs	nerve guidance conduits
NGF	nerve growth factor
OM-MSCs	olfactory mucosa mesenchymal stem cell
PCL	poly(D,L-lactide-co-ε-caprolactone)
PGA	poly(glycolic acid)
PGA	polyglycolic acid
PL	print length
PLA	poly(lactic acid)
PLF	print length factor

PLGA	poly(lactic-co-glycolic acid)
PNI	peripheral nerve injury
pRb	retinoblastoma gene product
PVA	polyvinyl alcohol
SFI	sciatic functional index
SSI	static sciatic index
TS	toe spread
TSF	toe spread factor
WJMSCs	Wharton's jelly mesenchymal stem cells
WRL	withdrawal reflex latency

Author details

Rui Damásio Alvites[1,2], Mariana Vieira Branquinho[1,2], Ana Rita Caseiro[1,2,3], Sílvia Santos Pedrosa[1,2], Ana Lúcia Luís[1,2], Stefano Geuna[4], Artur Severo Proença Varejão[5,6] and Ana Colette Maurício[1,2]*

1 Departamento de Clínicas Veterinárias, Instituto de Ciências Biomédicas de Abel Salazar (ICBAS), Universidade do Porto (UP), Porto, Portugal

2 Centro de Estudos de Ciência Animal (CECA), Instituto de Ciências, Tecnologias e Agroambiente da Universidade do Porto (ICETA), Porto, Portugal

3 Escola Universitária Vasco da Gama (EUVG), Coimbra, Portugal

4 Department of Clinical and Biological Sciences, Cavalieri Ottolenghi Neuroscience Institute, University of Turin, Turin, Italy

5 Departamento de Ciências Veterinárias, Universidade de Trás-os-Montes e Alto Douro (UTAD), Vila Real, Portugal

6 CECAV, Centro de Ciência Animal e Veterinária, Universidade de Trás-os-Montes e Alto Douro (UTAD), Vila Real, Portugal

*Address all correspondence to: ana.colette@hotmail.com

References

[1] Fathi SS, Zaminy A. Stem cell therapy for nerve injury. World Journal of Stem Cells. 2017;**9**(9):144

[2] Sullivan R, Dailey T, Duncan K, Abel N, Borlongan CV. Peripheral nerve injury: Stem cell therapy and peripheral nerve transfer. International Journal of Molecular Sciences. 2016;**17**(12):2101

[3] Taylor CA, Braza D, Rice JB, Dillingham T. The incidence of peripheral nerve injury in extremity trauma. American Journal of Physical Medicine & Rehabilitation. 2008;**87**(5):381-385

[4] Noble J, Munro CA, Prasad VS, Midha R. Analysis of upper and lower extremity peripheral nerve injuries in a population of patients with multiple injuries. Journal of Trauma and Acute Care Surgery. 1998;**45**(1):116-122

[5] Zhang X, Chen WW, Huang WJ. Chemotherapy-induced peripheral neuropathy. Biomedical Reports. 2017;**6**(3):267-271

[6] Pradat P-F, Delanian S. Late radiation injury to peripheral nerves. In: Handbook of Clinical Neurology. Vol. 115. Netherlands: Elsevier; 2013. pp. 743-758. DOI: 10.1016/B978-0-444-52902-2.00043-6

[7] Schreiber AK, Nones CF, Reis RC, Chichorro JG, Cunha JM. Diabetic neuropathic pain: Physiopathology and treatment. World Journal of Diabetes. 2015;**6**(3):432

[8] Antoine J-C, Camdessanché J-P. Peripheral nervous system involvement in patients with cancer. The Lancet Neurology. 2007;**6**(1):75-86

[9] Rasulić L, Savić A, Vitošević F, Samardžić M, Živković B, Mićović M, et al. Iatrogenic peripheral nerve injuries—Surgical treatment and outcome: 10 years' experience. World Neurosurgery. 2017;**103**:841-51.e6

[10] Antoniadis G. The peripheral nerve: Neuroanatomical principles before and after injury. In: Modern Concepts of Peripheral Nerve Repair. Unites States: Springer International Publishing; 2017. pp. 1-10. DOI: 10.1007/978-3-319-52319-4_1

[11] Catala M, Kubis N. Gross anatomy and development of the peripheral nervous system. In: Handbook of Clinical Neurology. Vol. 115. Netherlands: Elsevier; 2013. pp. 29-41. DOI: 10.1016/B978-0-444-52902-2.00003-5

[12] Pereira JA, Lebrun-Julien F, Suter U. Molecular mechanisms regulating myelination in the peripheral nervous system. Trends in Neurosciences. 2012;**35**(2):123-134

[13] Mizisin AP, Weerasuriya A. Homeostatic regulation of the endoneurial microenvironment during development, aging and in response to trauma, disease and toxic insult. Acta Neuropathologica. 2011;**121**(3):291-312

[14] Piña-Oviedo S, Ortiz-Hidalgo C. The normal and neoplastic perineurium: A review. Advances in Anatomic Pathology. 2008;**15**(3):147-164

[15] Lundborg G, Rydevik B. Effects of stretching the tibial nerve of the rabbit. A preliminary study of the intraneural circulation and the barrier function of the perineurium. Journal of Bone and Joint Surgery. 1973;**55**(2):390-401

[16] Peltonen S, Alanne M, Peltonen J. Barriers of the peripheral nerve. Tissue Barriers. 2013;**1**(3):e24956

[17] Olsson Y. Studies on vascular permeability in peripheral nerves. I.

Distribution of circulating fluorescent serum albumin in normal, crushed and sectioned rat sciatic nerve. Acta Neuropathologica. 1966;7(1):1-15

[18] Burnett MG, Zager EL. Pathophysiology of peripheral nerve injury: A brief review. Neurosurgical Focus. 2004;**16**(5):1-7

[19] Hainline BW. Peripheral nerve injury in sports. CONTINUUM: Lifelong Learning in Neurology. 2014;**20**(6, Sports Neurology):1605-1628

[20] Lim TK, Shi XQ, Johnson JM, Rone MB, Antel JP, David S, et al. Peripheral nerve injury induces persistent vascular dysfunction and endoneurial hypoxia, contributing to the genesis of neuropathic pain. Journal of Neuroscience. 2015;**35**(8):3346-3359

[21] Navarro X. Functional evaluation of peripheral nerve regeneration and target reinnervation in animal models: A critical overview. European Journal of Neuroscience. 2016;**43**(3):271-286

[22] Seddon H. Three types of nerve injury. Brain. 1943;**66**(4):237-288

[23] Sunderland S. A classification of peripheral nerve injuries producing loss of function. Brain. 1951;**74**(4):491-516

[24] Mackinnon S, Dellon A. Diagnosis of nerve injury. In: Surgery of the Peripheral Nerve. New York: Thieme; 1988. pp. 74-79

[25] Lutz AB, Barres BA. Contrasting the glial response to axon injury in the central and peripheral nervous systems. Developmental Cell. 2014;**28**(1):7-17

[26] Faroni A, Mobasseri SA, Kingham PJ, Reid AJ. Peripheral nerve regeneration: Experimental strategies and future perspectives. Advanced Drug Delivery Reviews. 2015;**82**:160-167

[27] Scheib J, Höke A. Advances in peripheral nerve regeneration. Nature Reviews Neurology. 2013;**9**(12):668

[28] Jonsson S, Wiberg R, McGrath AM, Novikov LN, Wiberg M, Novikova LN, et al. Effect of delayed peripheral nerve repair on nerve regeneration, Schwann cell function and target muscle recovery. PloS One. 2013;**8**(2):e56484

[29] Walsh S, Midha R. Practical considerations concerning the use of stem cells for peripheral nerve repair. Neurosurgical Focus. 2009;**26**(2):E2

[30] Alvites RD, Santos ARC, Varejão ASP, de Castro Osório ACP. Olfactory mucosa mesenchymal stem cells and biomaterials: A new combination to regenerative therapies after peripheral nerve injury. Mesenchymal Stem Cells-Isolation, Characterization and Applications: Rijeka InTech; 2017

[31] Carroll S, Worley S. Wallerian degeneration. In: Reference Module in Neuroscience and Biobehavioral Psychology. Netherlands: Elsevier; 2017. pp. 1-8. DOI: 10.1016/B978-0-12-809324-5.02077-0

[32] Hall S. The response to injury in the peripheral nervous system. The Journal of Bone and Joint Surgery British Volume. 2005;**87**(10):1309-1319

[33] Waller AV. Experiments on the section of the glossopharyngeal and hypoglossal nerves of the frog, and observations of the alterations produced thereby in the structure of their primitive fibres. Philosophical Transactions of the Royal Society of London. 1850;**140**:423-429

[34] Dubový P, Klusáková I Hradilová SI. Inflammatory profiling of Schwann cells in contact with growing axons distal to nerve injury. BioMed Research International. 2014;(7):1-7. DOI: 10.1155/2014/691041

[35] Perrin FE, Lacroix S, Avilés-Trigueros M, David S. Involvement of monocyte chemoattractant protein-1, macrophage inflammatory protein-1α and interleukin-1β in Wallerian degeneration. Brain. 2005;**128**(4):854-866

[36] Geuna S, Raimondo S, Ronchi G, Di Scipio F, Tos P, Czaja K, et al. Histology of the peripheral nerve and changes occurring during nerve regeneration. International Review of Neurobiology. 2009;**87**:27-46

[37] Menorca RM, Fussell TS, Elfar JC. Peripheral nerve trauma: Mechanisms of injury and recovery. Hand Clinics. 2013;**29**(3):317

[38] Deumens R, Bozkurt A, Meek MF, Marcus MA, Joosten EA, Weis J, et al. Repairing injured peripheral nerves: Bridging the gap. Progress in Neurobiology. 2010;**92**(3):245-276

[39] Alvites R, Rita Caseiro A, Santos Pedrosa S, Vieira Branquinho M, Ronchi G, Geuna S, et al. Peripheral nerve injury and axonotmesis: State of the art and recent advances. Cogent Medicine. 2018;**5**(1):1466404

[40] Houschyar K, Momeni A, Pyles M, Cha J, Maan Z, Duscher D, et al. The role of current techniques and concepts in peripheral nerve repair. Plastic Surgery International. 2016;**2016**:1-8. DOI: 10.1155/2016/4175293

[41] Au NPB, Kumar G, Asthana P, Tin C, Mak YL, Chan LL, et al. Ciguatoxin reduces regenerative capacity of axotomized peripheral neurons and delays functional recovery in pre-exposed mice after peripheral nerve injury. Scientific Reports. 2016;**6**:26809

[42] Trojaborg W. Rate of recovery in motor and sensory fibres of the radial nerve: Clinical and electrophysiological aspects. Journal of Neurology, Neurosurgery & Psychiatry. 1970;**33**(5):625-638

[43] Gaudet AD, Popovich PG, Ramer MS. Wallerian degeneration: Gaining perspective on inflammatory events after peripheral nerve injury. Journal of Neuroinflammation. 2011;**8**(1):110

[44] Höke A. Mechanisms of disease: What factors limit the success of peripheral nerve regeneration in humans? Nature Reviews Neurology. 2006;**2**(8):448

[45] Saied A, Shekaari MA, Sadeghifar A, Karbalaeikhani A. Introduction of a new suture method in repair of peripheral nerves injured with a sharp mechanism. Archives of Bone and Joint Surgery. 2015;**3**(4):254

[46] Dahlin L. Techniques of peripheral nerve repair. Scandinavian Journal of Surgery. 2008;**97**(4):310-316

[47] Peripheral nerve reconstruction after injury: A review of clinical and experimental therapies. BioMed Research International. 2014;**2014**:1-13. DOI: 10.1155/2014/698256

[48] Jerome JTJ. Anterior deltopectoral approach for axillary nerve neurotisation. Journal of Orthopaedic Surgery. 2012;**20**(1):66-70

[49] Rohde RS, Wolfe SW. Nerve transfers for adult traumatic brachial plexus palsy (brachial plexus nerve transfer). HSS Journal. 2007;**3**(1):77-82

[50] Simon NG, Spinner RJ, Kline DG, Kliot M. Advances in the neurological and neurosurgical management of peripheral nerve trauma. Journal of Neurology, Neurosurgery, and Psychiatry. 2016;**87**(2):198-208

[51] Matsuyama T, Mackay M, Midha R. Peripheral nerve repair and grafting techniques: A review.

Neurologia Medico-chirurgica. 2000;**40**(4):187-199

[52] Lundborg G. Bridging nerve defects-the role of tissue interpositioning. In: Severe Traumatic Defects of the Upper Limb. USA: CRC Press; 2004. pp. 151-165

[53] Millesi H. Bridging defects: Autologous nerve grafts. In: Acta Neurochir Suppl. Vol. 100. Austria: Springer-Verlag; 2007. pp. 37-38. DOI: 10.1007/978-3-211-72958-8_8

[54] Grand AG, Myckatyn TM, Mackinnon SE, Hunter DA. Axonal regeneration after cold preservation of nerve allografts and immunosuppression with tacrolimus in mice. Journal of Neurosurgery. 2002;**96**(5):924-932

[55] Safa B, Buncke G. Autograft substitutes: Conduits and processed nerve allografts. Hand Clinics. 2016;**32**(2):127-140

[56] Yi J-S, Lee H-J, Lee H-J, Lee I-W, Yang J-H. Rat peripheral nerve regeneration using nerve guidance channel by porcine small intestinal submucosa. Journal of Korean Neurosurgical Society. 2013;**53**(2):65

[57] Madduri S, Feldman K, Tervoort T, Papaloïzos M, Gander B. Collagen nerve conduits releasing the neurotrophic factors GDNF and NGF. Journal of Controlled Release. 2010;**143**(2):168-174

[58] Kehoe S, Zhang X, Boyd D. FDA approved guidance conduits and wraps for peripheral nerve injury: A review of materials and efficacy. Injury. 2012;**43**(5):553-572

[59] Babu P, Behl A, Chakravarty B, Bhandari P, Bhatti T, Maurya S. Entubulation techniques in peripheral nerve repair. Indian Journal of Neurotrauma. 2008;**5**(01):15-20

[60] Muheremu A, Ao Q. Past, present, and future of nerve conduits in the treatment of peripheral nerve injury. BioMed Research International. 2015;**2015**:237507

[61] Daly W, Yao L, Zeugolis D, Windebank A, Pandit A. A biomaterials approach to peripheral nerve regeneration: Bridging the peripheral nerve gap and enhancing functional recovery. Journal of the Royal Society Interface. 2012;**9**(67):202-221

[62] Pettersson J, McGrath A, Kalbermatten DF, Novikova LN, Wiberg M, Kingham PJ, et al. Muscle recovery after repair of short and long peripheral nerve gaps using fibrin conduits. Neuroscience Letters. 2011;**500**(1):41-46

[63] Simões MJ, Amado S, Gärtner A, Armada-da-Silva PA, Raimondo S, Vieira M, et al. Use of chitosan scaffolds for repairing rat sciatic nerve defects. Italian Journal of Anatomy and Embryology. 2010;**115**(3):190-210

[64] Scatena M, Eaton KV, Jackson MF, Lund SA, Giachelli CM. Macrophages: The bad, the ugly, and the good in the inflammatory response to biomaterials. In: The Immune Response to Implanted Materials and Devices. Switzerland: Springer International Publishing; 2017. pp. 37-62. DOI: 10.1007/978-3-319-45433-7_3

[65] Nectow AR, Marra KG, Kaplan DL. Biomaterials for the development of peripheral nerve guidance conduits. Tissue Engineering Part B: Reviews. 2011;**18**(1):40-50

[66] Basu B. Corrosion and degradation of implantable biomaterials. In: Biomaterials for Musculoskeletal Regeneration. Singapore: Springer Nature; 2017. pp. 253-289. DOI: 10.1007/978-981-10-3059-8_8

[67] Belanger K, Dinis TM, Taourirt S, Vidal G, Kaplan DL, Egles C. Recent strategies in tissue engineering for guided peripheral nerve regeneration. Macromolecular Bioscience. 2016;**16**(4):472-481

[68] Meek MF, Coert JH. US Food and Drug Administration/Conformit Europe-approved absorbable nerve conduits for clinical repair of peripheral and cranial nerves. Annals of Plastic Surgery. 2008;**60**(1):110-116

[69] Peng S-W, Li C-W, Chiu M, Wang G-J. Nerve guidance conduit with a hybrid structure of a PLGA microfibrous bundle wrapped in a micro/nanostructured membrane. International Journal of Nanomedicine. 2017;**12**:421

[70] Kaur G. Biomaterials influencing human lives. In: Bioactive Glasses. Switzerland: Springer International Publishing; 2017. pp. 1-20. DOI: 10.1007/978-3-319-45716-1_1

[71] Kokai LE, Lin Y-C, Oyster NM, Marra KG. Diffusion of soluble factors through degradable polymer nerve guides: Controlling manufacturing parameters. Acta Biomaterialia. 2009;**5**(7):2540-2550

[72] Xu J, Varitimidis SE, Fisher KJ, Tomaino MM, Sotereanos DG. The effect of wrapping scarred nerves with autogenous vein graft to treat recurrent chronic nerve compression. The Journal of Hand Surgery. 2000;**25**(1):93-103

[73] Suematsu N. Tubulation for peripheral nerve gap: Its history and possibility. Microsurgery. 1989;**10**(1):71-74

[74] Boyd JG, Gordon T. Neurotrophic factors and their receptors in axonal regeneration and functional recovery after peripheral nerve injury. Molecular Neurobiology. 2003;**27**(3):277-323

[75] Gaudin R, Knipfer C, Henningsen A, Smeets R, Heiland M, Hadlock T. Approaches to peripheral nerve repair: Generations of biomaterial conduits yielding to replacing autologous nerve grafts in craniomaxillofacial surgery. BioMed Research International. 2016;**2016**:1-18. DOI: 10.1155/2016/3856262

[76] Sariguney Y, Yavuzer R, Elmas C, Yenicesu I, Bolay H, Atabay K. Effect of platelet-rich plasma on peripheral nerve regeneration. Journal of Reconstructive Microsurgery. 2008;**24**(03):159-167

[77] Orbay H, Uysal AC, Hyakusoku H, Mizuno H. Differentiated and undifferentiated adipose-derived stem cells improve function in rats with peripheral nerve gaps. Journal of Plastic, Reconstructive & Aesthetic Surgery. 2012;**65**(5):657-664

[78] Hood B, Levene HB, Levi AD. Transplantation of autologous Schwann cells for the repair of segmental peripheral nerve defects. Neurosurgical Focus. 2009;**26**(2):E4

[79] Gao F, Chiu S, Motan D, Zhang Z, Chen L, Ji H, et al. Mesenchymal stem cells and immunomodulation: Current status and future prospects. Cell Death & Disease. 2017;7(1):e2062

[80] Al-Zer H, Kalbouneh H. Dental pulp stem cells-derived schwann cells for peripheral nerve injury regeneration. Neural Regeneration Research. 2015;**10**(12):1945

[81] Ge L, Jiang M, Duan D, Wang Z, Qi L, Teng X, et al. Secretome of olfactory mucosa mesenchymal stem cell, a multiple potential stem cell. Stem Cells International. 2016;**2016**:1-16. DOI: 10.1155/2016/1243659

[82] Talwadekar MD, Kale VP, Limaye LS. Placenta-derived mesenchymal stem cells possess better

immunoregulatory properties compared to their cord-derived counterparts—A paired sample study. Scientific Reports. 2015;**5**:15784

[83] Watson N, Divers R, Kedar R, Mehindru A, Mehindru A, Borlongan MC, et al. Discarded Wharton jelly of the human umbilical cord: A viable source for mesenchymal stromal cells. Cytotherapy. 2015;**17**(1):18-24

[84] Dominici M, Le Blanc K, Mueller I, Slaper-Cortenbach I, Marini F, Krause D, et al. Minimal criteria for defining multipotent mesenchymal stromal cells. The International Society for Cellular Therapy position statement. Cytotherapy. 2006;**8**(4):315-317

[85] Bhangra KS, Busuttil F, Phillips JB, Rahim AA. Using stem cells to grow artificial tissue for peripheral nerve repair. Stem Cells International. 2016;**2016**:1-18. DOI: 10.1155/2016/7502178

[86] Lalu MM, McIntyre L, Pugliese C, Fergusson D, Winston BW, Marshall JC, et al. Safety of cell therapy with mesenchymal stromal cells (SafeCell): A systematic review and meta-analysis of clinical trials. PLoS One. 2012;**7**(10):e47559

[87] Ankrum JA, Ong JF, Karp JM. Mesenchymal stem cells: Immune evasive, not immune privileged. Nature Biotechnology. 2014;**32**(3):252

[88] Grinnemo KH, Mansson A, Dellgren G, Klingberg D, Wardell E, Drvota V, et al. Xenoreactivity and engraftment of human mesenchymal stem cells transplanted into infarcted rat myocardium. Journal of Thoracic and Cardiovascular Surgery. 2004;**127**(5):1293-1300

[89] Xia Z, Ye H, Choong C, Ferguson DJ, Platt N, Cui Z, et al. Macrophagic response to human mesenchymal stem cell and poly(epsilon-caprolactone) implantation in nonobese diabetic/severe combined immunodeficient mice. Journal of Biomedical Materials Research Part A. 2004;**71**(3):538-548

[90] Moll G, Rasmusson-Duprez I, von Bahr L, Connolly-Andersen AM, Elgue G, Funke L, et al. Are therapeutic human mesenchymal stromal cells compatible with human blood? Stem Cells. 2012;**30**(7):1565-1574

[91] Pig J, Ishihara A, Wellman ML, Russell DS, Bertone A. Inflammatory effects of autologous, genetically modified autologous, allogeneic, and xenogeneic mesenchymal stem cells after intra-articular injection in horses. Veterinary and Comparative Orthopaedics and Traumatology. 2013;**26**(06):453-460

[92] Joswig AJ, Mitchell A, Cummings KJ, Levine GJ, Gregory CA, Smith R 3rd, et al. Repeated intra-articular injection of allogeneic mesenchymal stem cells causes an adverse response compared to autologous cells in the equine model. Stem Cell Research & Therapy. 2017;**8**(1):42

[93] Von Bahr L, Batsis I, Moll G, Hägg M, Szakos A, Sundberg B, et al. Analysis of tissues following mesenchymal stromal cell therapy in humans indicates limited long-term engraftment and no ectopic tissue formation. Stem Cells. 2012;**30**(7):1575-1578

[94] Kingham PJ, Kalbermatten DF, Mahay D, Armstrong SJ, Wiberg M, Terenghi G. Adipose-derived stem cells differentiate into a Schwann cell phenotype and promote neurite outgrowth in vitro. Experimental Neurology. 2007;**207**(2):267-274

[95] Keilhoff G, Goihl A, Langnase K, Fansa H, Wolf G. Transdifferentiation of mesenchymal stem cells into Schwann cell-like myelinating cells. European Journal of Cell Biology. 2006;**85**(1):11-24

[96] Zaminy A, Shokrgozar MA, Sadeghi Y, Noroozian M, Heidari MH, Piryaei A. Mesenchymal stem cells as an alternative for Schwann cells in rat spinal cord injury. Iranian Biomedical Journal. 2013;**17**(3):113

[97] Cj P, Tong L, Ll J, Wang Z, Zhang X, Gao H, et al. Synergistic effects of ultrashort wave and bone marrow stromal cells on nerve regeneration with acellular nerve allografts. Synapse. 2013;**67**(10):637-647

[98] Zhao Z, Wang Y, Peng J, Ren Z, Zhang L, Guo Q, et al. Improvement in nerve regeneration through a decellularized nerve graft by supplementation with bone marrow stromal cells in fibrin. Cell Transplantation. 2014;**23**(1):97-110

[99] Shalaby SM, Amal S, Ahmed FE, Shaban SF, Wahdan RA, Kandel WA, et al. Combined Wharton's jelly derived mesenchymal stem cells and nerve guidance conduit: A potential promising therapy for peripheral nerve injuries. The International Journal of Biochemistry & Cell Biology. 2017;**86**:67-76

[100] Schmidt CE, Leach JB. Neural tissue engineering: Strategies for repair and regeneration. Annual Review of Biomedical Engineering. 2003;**5**(1):293-347

[101] Tabesh H, Amoabediny G, Nik NS, Heydari M, Yosefifard M, Siadat SR, et al. The role of biodegradable engineered scaffolds seeded with Schwann cells for spinal cord regeneration. Neurochemistry International. 2009;**54**(2):73-83

[102] Deshmukh SN, Dive AM, Moharil R, Munde P. Enigmatic insight into collagen. Journal of Oral and Maxillofacial Pathology: JOMFP. 2016;**20**(2):276

[103] Brown R, Alovskaya A, Alekseeva T, Phillips J, King V. Fibronectin, collagen, fibrincompnents of extracellular matrix for nerve regeneration. In: Topics in Tissue Engineering. Vol. 3. Finland: Oulu University; 2007. pp. 1-26

[104] Amado S, Rodrigues JM, Luís AL, Armada-da-Silva PA, Vieira M, Gartner A, et al. Effects of collagen membranes enriched with in vitro-differentiated N1E-115 cells on rat sciatic nerve regeneration after end-to-end repair. Journal of Neuroengineering and Rehabilitation. 2010;**7**(1):7

[105] Brown RA, Phillips JB. Cell responses to biomimetic protein scaffolds used in tissue repair and engineering. International Review of Cytology. 2007;**262**:75-150

[106] Yoshii S, Oka M. Peripheral nerve regeneration along collagen filaments. Brain Research. 2001;**888**(1):158-162

[107] Phillips JB, Bunting SC, Hall SM, Brown RA. Neural tissue engineering: A self-organizing collagen guidance conduit. Tissue Engineering. 2005;**11**(9-10):1611-1617

[108] Ceballos D, Navarro X, Dubey N, Wendelschafer-Crabb G, Kennedy WR, Tranquillo RT. Magnetically aligned collagen gel filling a collagen nerve guide improves peripheral nerve regeneration. Experimental Neurology. 1999;**158**(2):290-300

[109] Chamberlain LJ, Yannas IV, Hsu HP, Spector M. Connective tissue response to tubular implants for peripheral nerve regeneration: The role of myofibroblasts. Journal of Comparative Neurology. 2000;**417**(4):415-430

[110] Archibald SJ, Krarup C, Shefner J, Li ST, Madison RD. A collagen-based nerve guide conduit for peripheral nerve repair: An electrophysiological study of nerve regeneration in rodents and nonhuman primates. Journal of Comparative Neurology. 1991;**306**(4):685-696

[111] Luís A, Rodrigues J, Geuna S, Amado S, Simões M, Fregnan F, et al. Neural cell transplantation effects on sciatic nerve regeneration after a standardized crush injury in the rat. Microsurgery: Official Journal of the International Microsurgical Society and the European Federation of Societies for Microsurgery. 2008;**28**(6):458-470

[112] Mackinnon SE, Hudson AR, Bojanowski V, Hunter DA, Maraghi E. Peripheral nerve injection injury with purified bovine collagen—An experimental model in the rat. Annals of Plastic Surgery. 1985;**14**(5):428-436

[113] Kramer BA, Kadar AG, Clark K. Use of the Neuro-Wrap system for severe post-electroconvulsive therapy headaches. The Journal of ECT. 2008;**24**(2):152-155

[114] Li S-T, Yuen D. Implant devices for nerve repair. Google Patents; 2004

[115] Lohmeyer JA, Siemers F, Machens H-G, Mailänder P. The clinical use of artificial nerve conduits for digital nerve repair: A prospective cohort study and literature review. Journal of Reconstructive Microsurgery. 2009;**25**(01):055-061

[116] Salvatore L, Madaghiele M, Parisi C, Gatti F, Sannino A. Crosslinking of micropatterned collagen-based nerve guides to modulate the expected half-life. Journal of Biomedical Materials Research Part A. 2014;**102**(12):4406-4414

[117] Yang CR, Di Chen J. Preparation and biological evaluation of chitosan–collagen–icariin composite scaffolds for neuronal regeneration. Neurological Sciences. 2013;**34**(6):941-947

[118] Cerri F, Salvatore L, Memon D, Boneschi FM, Madaghiele M, Brambilla P, et al. Peripheral nerve morphogenesis induced by scaffold micropatterning. Biomaterials. 2014;**35**(13):4035-4045

[119] Bąk M, Gutkowska O, Wagner E, Gosk J. The role of chitin and chitosan in peripheral nerve reconstruction. Polimery w Medycynie. 2017;**47**(1):43-47

[120] Lu G, Kong L, Sheng B, Wang G, Gong Y, Zhang X. Degradation of covalently cross-linked carboxymethyl chitosan and its potential application for peripheral nerve regeneration. European Polymer Journal. 2007;**43**(9):3807-3818

[121] Freier T, Koh HS, Kazazian K, Shoichet MS. Controlling cell adhesion and degradation of chitosan films by N-acetylation. Biomaterials. 2005;**26**(29):5872-5878

[122] Freier T, Montenegro R, Koh HS, Shoichet MS. Chitin-based tubes for tissue engineering in the nervous system. Biomaterials. 2005;**26**(22):4624-4632

[123] Wang W, Itoh S, Matsuda A, Ichinose S, Shinomiya K, Hata Y, et al. Influences of mechanical properties and permeability on chitosan nano/microfiber mesh tubes as a scaffold for nerve regeneration. Journal of Biomedical Materials Research Part A. 2008;**84**(2):557-566

[124] Shirosaki Y, Hayakawa S, Osaka A, Lopes MA, Santos JD, Geuna S, et al. Challenges for nerve repair using chitosan-siloxane hybrid porous scaffolds. BioMed Research

International. 2014;**2014**:1-7. DOI: 10.1155/2014/153808

[125] Wang W, Itoh S, Matsuda A, Aizawa T, Demura M, Ichinose S, et al. Enhanced nerve regeneration through a bilayered chitosan tube: The effect of introduction of glycine spacer into the CYIGSR sequence. Journal of Biomedical Materials Research Part A: An Official Journal of the Society for Biomaterials, The Japanese Society for Biomaterials, and the Australian Society for Biomaterials and the Korean Society for Biomaterials. 2008;**85**(4):919-928

[126] Szymańska E, Winnicka K. Stability of chitosan—A challenge for pharmaceutical and biomedical applications. Marine Drugs. 2015;**13**(4):1819-1846

[127] Mingyu C, Kai G, Jiamou L, Yandao G, Nanming Z, Xiufang Z. Surface modification and characterization of chitosan film blended with poly-L-lysine. Journal of Biomaterials Applications. 2004;**19**(1):59-75

[128] Cheng M, Deng J, Yang F, Gong Y, Zhao N, Zhang X. Study on physical properties and nerve cell affinity of composite films from chitosan and gelatin solutions. Biomaterials. 2003;**24**(17):2871-2880

[129] Wang X, Hu W, Cao Y, Yao J, Wu J, Gu X. Dog sciatic nerve regeneration across a 30-mm defect bridged by a chitosan/PGA artificial nerve graft. Brain. 2005;**128**(8):1897-1910

[130] Gärtner A, Pereira T, Simões MJ, Armada-da-Silva PA, França ML, Sousa R, et al. Use of hybrid chitosan membranes and human mesenchymal stem cells from the Wharton jelly of umbilical cord for promoting nerve regeneration in an axonotmesis rat model. Neural Regeneration Research. 2012;**7**(29):2247

[131] Itoh S, Suzuki M, Yamaguchi I, Takakuda K, Kobayashi H, Shinomiya K, et al. Development of a nerve scaffold using a tendon chitosan tube. Artificial Organs. 2003;**27**(12):1079-1088

[132] Lin Y-L, Jen J-C, Hsu S-H, Chiu M. Sciatic nerve repair by microgrooved nerve conduits made of chitosan-gold nanocomposites. Surgical Neurology. 2008;**70**:S9-S18

[133] Haastert-Talini K, Geuna S, Dahlin LB, Meyer C, Stenberg L, Freier T, et al. Chitosan tubes of varying degrees of acetylation for bridging peripheral nerve defects. Biomaterials. 2013;**34**(38):9886-9904

[134] Gonzalez-Perez F, Cobianchi S, Geuna S, Barwig C, Freier T, Udina E, et al. Tubulization with chitosan guides for the repair of long gap peripheral nerve injury in the rat. Microsurgery. 2015;**35**(4):300-308

[135] Baldrick P. The safety of chitosan as a pharmaceutical excipient. Regulatory Toxicology and Pharmacology. 2010;**56**(3):290-299

[136] Patel M, Mao L, Wu B, VandeVord PJ. GDNF–chitosan blended nerve guides: A functional study. Journal of Tissue Engineering and Regenerative Medicine. 2007;**1**(5):360-367

[137] Boucher TJ, Okuse K, Bennett DL, Munson JB, Wood JN, McMahon SB. Potent analgesic effects of GDNF in neuropathic pain states. Science. 2000;**290**(5489):124-127

[138] Hsu S-H, Kuo W-C, Chen Y-T, Yen C-T, Chen Y-F, Chen K-S, et al. New nerve regeneration strategy combining laminin-coated chitosan conduits and stem cell therapy. Acta Biomaterialia. 2013;**9**(5):6606-6615

[139] Lauto A, Foster LJ, Avolio A, Sampson D, Raston C, Sarris M, et al.

Sutureless nerve repair with laser-activated chitosan adhesive: A pilot in vivo study. Photomedicine and Laser Surgery. 2008;**26**(3):227-234

[140] Cortez P, Shirosaki Y, Botelho C, Simões M, Gartner F, da Costa R, et al. Hybrid chitosan membranes tested in sheep for guided tissue regeneration. In: Key Engineering Materials. Vols. 361-363. Switzerland: Trans Tech Publications; 2008. pp. 1265-1268. DOI: 10.4028/www.scientific.net/KEM.361-363.1265

[141] Shirosaki Y, Hayakawa S, Osaka A, Santos JD, Maurício AC. Nerve regeneration by using of chitosansilicate hybrid porous membranes. In: Key Engineering Materials. Vols. 529-530(1). Switzerland: Trans Tech Publications; 2013. pp. 361-364. DOI: 10.4028/www.scientific.net/KEM.529-530.361

[142] Shirosaki Y, Tsuru K, Hayakawa S, Osaka A, Lopes MA, Santos JD, et al. In vitro cytocompatibility of MG63 cells on chitosan-organosiloxane hybrid membranes. Biomaterials. 2005;**26**(5):485-493

[143] Shirosaki Y, Tsuru K, Hayakawa S, Osaka A, Lopes MA, Santos JD, et al. Physical, chemical and in vitro biological profile of chitosan hybrid membrane as a function of organosiloxane concentration. Acta Biomaterialia. 2009;**5**(1):346-355

[144] Amado S, Simoes M, da Silva PA, Luís A, Shirosaki Y, Lopes M, et al. Use of hybrid chitosan membranes and N1E-115 cells for promoting nerve regeneration in an axonotmesis rat model. Biomaterials. 2008;**29**(33):4409-4419

[145] Tateishi T, Chen G, Ushida T. Biodegradable porous scaffolds for tissue engineering. Journal of Artificial Organs. 2002;**5**(2):77-83

[146] Shirosaki Y, Okayama T, Tsuru K, Hayakawa S, Osaka A. Synthesis and cytocompatibility of porous chitosan–silicate hybrids for tissue engineering scaffold application. Chemical Engineering Journal. 2008;**137**(1):122-128

[147] Simoes M, Gärtner A, Shirosaki Y, da Costa RG, Cortez P, Gartner F, et al. In vitro and in vivo chitosan membranes testing for peripheral nerve reconstruction. Acta Medica Portuguesa. 2011;**24**(1):43-52

[148] Xynos ID, Edgar AJ, Buttery LD, Hench LL, Polak JM. Gene-expression profiling of human osteoblasts following treatment with the ionic products of Bioglass® 45S5 dissolution. Journal of Biomedical Materials Research: An Official Journal of The Society for Biomaterials, The Japanese Society for Biomaterials, and The Australian Society for Biomaterials and the Korean Society for Biomaterials. 2001;**55**(2):151-157

[149] Neubrech F, Heider S, Harhaus L, Bickert B, Kneser U, Kremer T. Chitosan nerve tube for primary repair of traumatic sensory nerve lesions of the hand without a gap: study protocol for a randomized controlled trial. Trials. 2016;**17**:48. DOI: 10.1186/s13063-015-1148-5

[150] Fornasari BE, Gambarotta G, Ronchi G, Raimondo S, Crosio A, Budau CA, et al. Chitosan tubes enriched by skeletal muscle for peripheral nerve regeneration. In: 6th Symposium on Surgery of Peripheral Nerves. 2017

[151] Willerth SM, Sakiyama-Elbert SE. Approaches to neural tissue engineering using scaffolds for drug delivery. Advanced Drug Delivery Reviews. 2007;**59**(4-5):325-338

[152] Dellon A, Chang B. An alternative incision for approaching recurrent

median nerve compression at the wrist. Plastic and Reconstructive Surgery. 1992;**89**(3):576-578

[153] Costa HJZR, Bento RF, Salomone R, Azzi-Nogueira D, Zanatta DB, Costa MP, et al. Mesenchymal bone marrow stem cells within polyglycolic acid tube observed in vivo after six weeks enhance facial nerve regeneration. Brain Research. 2013;**1510**:10-21

[154] Arslantunali D, Dursun T, Yucel D, Hasirci N, Hasirci V. Peripheral nerve conduits: Technology update. Medical Devices (Auckland, NZ). 2014;**7**:405

[155] Zhang Z, Ortiz O, Goyal R, Kohn J. Biodegradable polymers. In: Principles of Tissue Engineering. Netherlands: Elsevier; 2014. pp. 441-473. DOI: 10.1016/B978-0-12-398358-9.00023-9

[156] Lu M-C, Huang Y-T, Lin J-H, Yao C-H, Lou C-W, Tsai C-C, et al. Evaluation of a multi-layer microbraided polylactic acid fiber-reinforced conduit for peripheral nerve regeneration. Journal of Materials Science: Materials in Medicine. 2009;**20**(5):1175-1180

[157] S-h H, Chan S-H, Chiang C-M, Chen CC-C, Jiang C-F. Peripheral nerve regeneration using a microporous polylactic acid asymmetric conduit in a rabbit long-gap sciatic nerve transection model. Biomaterials. 2011;**32**(15):3764-3775

[158] Matsumine H, Sasaki R, Yamato M, Okano T, Sakurai H. A polylactic acid non-woven nerve conduit for facial nerve regeneration in rats. Journal of Tissue Engineering and Regenerative Medicine. 2014;**8**(6):454-462

[159] Ni H-C, Tseng T-C, Chen J-R, Hsu S-H, Chiu M. Fabrication of bioactive conduits containing the fibroblast growth factor 1 and neural stem cells for peripheral nerve regeneration across a 15 mm critical gap. Biofabrication. 2013;**5**(3):035010

[160] Reed A, Gilding D. Biodegradable polymers for use in surgery—Poly (glycolic)/poly (Iactic acid) homo and copolymers: 2. In vitro degradation. Polymer. 1981;**22**(4):494-498

[161] Oh SH, Lee JH. Fabrication and characterization of hydrophilized porous PLGA nerve guide conduits by a modified immersion precipitation method. Journal of Biomedical Materials Research Part A. 2007;**80**(3):530-538

[162] Lin K-M, Shea J, Gale BK, Sant H, Larrabee P, Agarwal J. Nerve growth factor released from a novel PLGA nerve conduit can improve axon growth. Journal of Micromechanics and Microengineering. 2016;**26**(4):045016

[163] Hadlock T, Sundback C, Hunter D, Cheney M, Vacanti JP. A polymer foam conduit seeded with Schwann cells promotes guided peripheral nerve regeneration. Tissue Engineering. 2000;**6**(2):119-127

[164] Pereira T, Gärtner A, Amorim I, Almeida A, Caseiro A, Armadada-Silva PA, et al. Promoting nerve regeneration in a neurotmesis rat model using poly(DL-lactide-caprolactone) membranes and mesenchymal stem cells from the Wharton's jelly: In vitro and in vivo analysis. BioMed Research International. 2014;**2014**:1-17. DOI: 10.1155/2014/302659

[165] Labroo P, Shea J, Edwards K, Ho S, Davis B, Sant H, et al. Novel drug delivering conduit for peripheral nerve regeneration. Journal of Neural Engineering. 2017;**14**(6):066011

[166] Doubra N, Amiri A, Jamalpoor Z, Fooladi AAI, Nourani MR. Fabrication of PLGA conduit for peripheral nerve regeneration. Journal of Applied Tissue Engineering. 2014;**1**(1):13-19

[167] Venugopal J, Zhang Y, Ramakrishna S. Electrospun nanofibres: Biomedical applications. Proceedings of the Institution of Mechanical Engineers, Part N: Journal of Nanoengineering and Nanosystems. 2004;**218**(1):35-45

[168] Radulescu D, Dhar S, Young CM, Taylor DW, Trost H-J, Hayes DJ, et al. Tissue engineering scaffolds for nerve regeneration manufactured by ink-jet technology. Materials Science and Engineering: C. 2007;**27**(3):534-539

[169] McConnell MP, Dhar S, Nguyen T, Naran S, Calvert JW, Sundine MJ, et al. Nerve growth factor expression response to induction agent booster dosing in transfected human embryonic kidney cells. Plastic and Reconstructive Surgery. 2005;**115**(2):506-514

[170] Luis AL, Rodrigues JM, Amado S, Veloso AP, Armada-Da-silva PA, Raimondo S, et al. PLGA 90/10 and caprolactone biodegradable nerve guides for the reconstruction of the rat sciatic nerve. Microsurgery: Official Journal of the International Microsurgical Society and the European Federation of Societies for Microsurgery. 2007;**27**(2):125-137

[171] Shin RH, Friedrich PF, Crum BA, Bishop AT, Shin AY. Treatment of a segmental nerve defect in the rat with use of bioabsorbable synthetic nerve conduits: A comparison of commercially available conduits. JBJS. 2009;**91**(9):2194-2204

[172] Chiriac S, Facca S, Diaconu M, Gouzou S, Liverneaux P. Experience of using the bioresorbable copolyester poly (DL-lactide-ε-caprolactone) nerve conduit guide Neurolac™ for nerve repair in peripheral nerve defects: Report on a series of 28 lesions. Journal of Hand Surgery (European Volume). 2012;**37**(4):342-349

[173] Grant C, Twigg P, Egan A, Moody A, Smith A, Eagland D, et al. Poly(vinyl alcohol) hydrogel as a biocompatible viscoelastic mimetic for articular cartilage. Biotechnology Progress. 2006;**22**(5):1400-1406

[174] Alexandre N, Amorim I, Caseiro AR, Pereira T, Alvites R, Rêma A, et al. Long term performance evaluation of small-diameter vascular grafts based on polyvinyl alcohol hydrogel and dextran and MSCs-based therapies using the ovine pre-clinical animal model. International Journal of Pharmaceutics. 2017;**523**(2):515-530

[175] Alexandre N, Costa E, Coimbra S, Silva A, Lopes A, Rodrigues M, et al. In vitro and in vivo evaluation of blood coagulation activation of polyvinyl alcohol hydrogel plus dextran-based vascular grafts. Journal of Biomedical Materials Research Part A. 2015;**103**(4):1366-1379

[176] Bichara DA, Zhao X, Hwang NS, Bodugoz-Senturk H, Yaremchuk MJ, Randolph MA, et al. Porous poly (vinyl alcohol)-alginate gel hybrid construct for neocartilage formation using human nasoseptal cells. Journal of Surgical Research. 2010;**163**(2):331-336

[177] Rutkowski GE, Heath CA. Development of a bioartificial nerve graft. II. Nerve regeneration in vitro. Biotechnology Progress. 2002;**18**(2):373-379

[178] Ribeiro J, Caseiro AR, Pereira T, Armada-da-Silva PA, Pires I, Prada J, et al. Evaluation of PVA biodegradable electric conductive membranes for nerve regeneration in axonotmesis injuries: The rat sciatic nerve animal model. Journal of Biomedical Materials Research Part A. 2017;**105**(5):1267-1280

[179] Ribeiro J, Pereira T, Caseiro AR, Armada-da-Silva P, Pires I, Prada J, et al.

Evaluation of biodegradable electric conductive tube-guides and mesenchymal stem cells. World Journal of Stem Cells. 2015;**7**(6):956

[180] Chen Z-L, Yu W-M, Strickland S. Peripheral regeneration. Annual Review of Neuroscience. 2007;**30**:209-233

[181] Amano T, Richelson E, Nirenberg M. Neurotransmitter synthesis by neuroblastoma clones. Proceedings of the National Academy of Sciences. 1972;**69**(1):258-263

[182] Kimhi Y, Palfrey C, Spector I, Barak Y, Littauer U. Maturation of neuroblastoma cells in the presence of dimethylsulfoxide. Proceedings of the National Academy of Sciences. 1976;**73**(2):462-466

[183] Prasad KN, Kentroti S, Edwards-Prasad J, Vernadakis A, Imam M, Carvalho E, et al. Modification of the expression of adenosine 3′,5′-cyclic monophosphate-induced differentiated functions in neuroblastoma cells by beta-carotene and D-alpha-tocopheryl succinate. Journal of the American College of Nutrition. 1994;**13**(3):298-303

[184] Rodrigues J, Luís A, Lobato J, Pinto M, Lopes M, Freitas M, et al. Determination of the intracellular Ca^{2+} concentration in the N1E-115 neuronal cell line in perspective of its use for peripheric nerve regeneration. Bio-medical Materials and Engineering. 2005;**15**(6):455-465

[185] Rodrigues J, Luís A, Lobato J, Pinto M, Faustino A, Hussain NS, et al. Intracellular Ca^{2+} concentration in the N1E-115 neuronal cell line and its use for peripheric nerve regeneration. Acta Médica Portuguesa. 2005;**18**(5):323-328

[186] Luís AL, Rodrigues JM, Geuna S, Amado S, Shirosaki Y, Lee JM, et al. Use of PLGA 90: 10 scaffolds enriched with in vitro–differentiated neural cells for repairing rat sciatic nerve defects. Tissue Engineering Part A. 2008;**14**(6):979-993

[187] Fairbairn N, Randolph M, Redmond R. The clinical applications of human amnion in plastic surgery. Journal of Plastic, Reconstructive & Aesthetic Surgery. 2014;**67**(5):662-675

[188] Fu YS, Cheng YC, Lin MYA, Cheng H, Chu PM, Chou SC, et al. Conversion of human umbilical cord mesenchymal stem cells in Wharton's jelly to dopaminergic neurons in vitro: Potential therapeutic application for Parkinsonism. Stem Cells. 2006;**24**(1):115-124

[189] Frausin S, Viventi S, Falzacappa LV, Quattromani MJ, Leanza G, Tommasini A, et al. Wharton's jelly derived mesenchymal stromal cells: Biological properties, induction of neuronal phenotype and current applications in neurodegeneration research. Acta Histochemica. 2015;**117**(4-5):329-338

[190] Gärtner A, Pereira T, Armada-da-Silva P, Amorim I, Gomes R, Ribeiro J, et al. Use of poly(DL-lactide-ε-caprolactone) membranes and mesenchymal stem cells from the Wharton's jelly of the umbilical cord for promoting nerve regeneration in axonotmesis: In vitro and in vivo analysis. Differentiation. 2012;**84**(5):355-365

[191] Cheng L-N, Duan X-H, Zhong X-M, Guo R-M, Zhang F, Zhou C-P, et al. Transplanted neural stem cells promote nerve regeneration in acute peripheral nerve traction injury: Assessment using MRI. American Journal of Roentgenology. 2011;**196**(6):1381-1387

[192] Jiang L, Jones S, Jia X. Stem cell transplantation for peripheral nerve regeneration: Current options and opportunities. International Journal of Molecular Sciences. 2017;**18**(1):94

[193] Caseiro AR, Pereira T, Ribeiro J, Amorim I, Faria F, Bártolo PJ, et al. Neuro-muscular regeneration using scaffolds with mesenchymal stem cells (MSCs) Isolated from human umbilical cord Wharton's jelly: Functional and morphological analysis using rat sciatic nerve neurotmesis injury model. Procedia Engineering. 2015;**110**:106-113

[194] Marcus AJ, Woodbury D. Fetal stem cells from extra-embryonic tissues: Do not discard. Journal of Cellular and Molecular Medicine. 2008;**12**(3):730-742

[195] Peng J, Wang Y, Zhang L, Zhao B, Zhao Z, Chen J, et al. Human umbilical cord Wharton's jelly-derived mesenchymal stem cells differentiate into a Schwann-cell phenotype and promote neurite outgrowth in vitro. Brain Research Bulletin. 2011;**84**(3):235-243

[196] Ribeiro J, Pereira T, Amorim I, Caseiro AR, Lopes MA, Lima J, et al. Cell therapy with human MSCs isolated from the umbilical cord Wharton jelly associated to a PVA membrane in the treatment of chronic skin wounds. International Journal of Medical Sciences. 2014;**11**(10):979

[197] Pereira T, Armada-da Silva P, Amorim I, Rêma A, Caseiro A, Gärtner A, et al. Effects of human mesenchymal stem cells isolated from Wharton's jelly of the umbilical cord and conditioned media on skeletal muscle regeneration using a myectomy model. Stem Cells International. 2014;**2014**:1-16. DOI: 10.1155/2014/376918

[198] Gärtner A, Pereira T, Armada-da-Silva P, Amado S, Veloso A, Amorim I, et al. Effects of umbilical cord tissue mesenchymal stem cells (UCX®) on rat sciatic nerve regeneration after neurotmesis injuries. Journal of Stem Cells & Regenerative Medicine. 2014;**10**(1):14

[199] Luo L, He Y, Wang X, Key B, Lee BH, Li H, et al. Potential roles of dental pulp stem cells in neural regeneration and repair. Stem Cells International. 2018;**2018**:1-15. DOI: 10.1155/2018/1731289

[200] Gronthos S, Mankani M, Brahim J, Robey PG, Shi S. Postnatal human dental pulp stem cells (DPSCs) in vitro and in vivo. Proceedings of the National Academy of Sciences. 2000;**97**(25):13625-13630

[201] Struillou X, Boutigny H, Soueidan A, Layrolle P. Experimental animal models in periodontology: A review. The Open Dentistry Journal. 2010;**4**:37

[202] Karbanová J, Soukup T, Suchánek J, Pytlík R, Corbeil D, Mokrý J. Characterization of dental pulp stem cells from impacted third molars cultured in low serum-containing medium. Cells Tissues Organs. 2011;**193**(6):344-365

[203] Gronthos S, Brahim J, Li W, Fisher L, Cherman N, Boyde A, et al. Stem cell properties of human dental pulp stem cells. Journal of Dental Research. 2002;**81**(8):531-535

[204] Kawashima N. Characterisation of dental pulp stem cells: A new horizon for tissue regeneration? Archives of Oral Biology. 2012;**57**(11):1439-1458

[205] Sakai K, Yamamoto A, Matsubara K, Nakamura S, Naruse M, Yamagata M, et al. Human dental pulp-derived stem cells promote locomotor recovery after complete transection of the rat spinal cord by multiple neuro-regenerative mechanisms. The Journal of Clinical Investigation. 2012;**122**(1):80-90

[206] Miura M, Gronthos S, Zhao M, Lu B, Fisher LW, Robey PG, et al. SHED: Stem cells from human exfoliated deciduous teeth. Proceedings of

the National Academy of Sciences. 2003;**100**(10):5807-5812

[207] Kiraly M, Porcsalmy B, Pataki A, Kadar K, Jelitai M, Molnar B, et al. Simultaneous PKC and cAMP activation induces differentiation of human dental pulp stem cells into functionally active neurons. Neurochemistry International. 2009;**55**(5):323-332

[208] Sugimura-Wakayama Y, Katagiri W, Osugi M, Kawai T, Ogata K, Sakaguchi K, et al. Peripheral nerve regeneration by secretomes of stem cells from human exfoliated deciduous teeth. Stem Cells and Development. 2015;**24**(22):2687-2699

[209] Askari N, Yaghoobi M, Shamsara M, Esmaeili-Mahani S. Tetracycline-regulated expression of OLIG2 gene in human dental pulp stem cells lead to mouse sciatic nerve regeneration upon transplantation. Neuroscience. 2015;**305**:197-208

[210] Geng YW, Zhang Z, Liu MY, Hu WP. Differentiation of human dental pulp stem cells into neuronal by resveratrol. Cell Biology International. 2017;**41**(12):1391-1398

[211] Arthur A, Shi S, Zannettino AC, Fujii N, Gronthos S, Koblar SA. Implanted adult human dental pulp stem cells induce endogenous axon guidance. Stem Cells. 2009;**27**(9):2229-2237

[212] Martens W, Sanen K, Georgiou M, Struys T, Bronckaers A, Ameloot M, et al. Human dental pulp stem cells can differentiate into Schwann cells and promote and guide neurite outgrowth in an aligned tissue-engineered collagen construct in vitro. The FASEB Journal. 2014;**28**(4):1634-1643

[213] Yamamoto T, Osako Y, Ito M, Murakami M, Hayashi Y, Horibe H, et al. Trophic effects of dental pulp stem cells on schwann cells in peripheral nerve regeneration. Cell Transplantation. 2016;**25**(1):183-193

[214] Potdar PD, Jethmalani YD. Human dental pulp stem cells: Applications in future regenerative medicine. World Journal of Stem Cells. 2015;**7**(5):839

[215] Sasaki R, Aoki S, Yamato M, Uchiyama H, Wada K, Okano T, et al. Tubulation with dental pulp cells promotes facial nerve regeneration in rats. Tissue Engineering Part A. 2008;**14**(7):1141-1147

[216] Sasaki R, Aoki S, Yamato M, Uchiyama H, Wada K, Ogiuchi H, et al. PLGA artificial nerve conduits with dental pulp cells promote facial nerve regeneration. Journal of Tissue Engineering and Regenerative Medicine. 2011;**5**(10):823-830

[217] Sanen K, Martens W, Georgiou M, Ameloot M, Lambrichts I, Phillips J. Engineered neural tissue with Schwann cell differentiated human dental pulp stem cells: Potential for peripheral nerve repair? Journal of Tissue Engineering and Regenerative Medicine. 2017;**11**(12):3362-3372

[218] Dai L-G, Huang G-S, S-h H. Sciatic nerve regeneration by cocultured Schwann cells and stem cells on microporous nerve conduits. Cell Transplantation. 2013;**22**(11):2029-2039

[219] Ullah I, Park J-M, Kang Y-H, Byun J-H, Kim D-G, Kim J-H, et al. Transplantation of human dental pulp-derived stem cells or differentiated neuronal cells from human dental pulp-derived stem cells identically enhances regeneration of the injured peripheral nerve. Stem Cells and Development. 2017;**26**(17):1247-1257

[220] Omi M, Hata M, Nakamura N, Miyabe M, Kobayashi Y, Kamiya H, et al. Transplantation of dental pulp stem cells suppressed inflammation in sciatic nerves by promoting macrophage

polarization towards anti-inflammation phenotypes and ameliorated diabetic polyneuropathy. Journal of Diabetes Investigation. 2016;7(4):485-496

[221] Delorme B, Nivet E, Gaillard J, Häupl T, Ringe J, Devèze A, et al. The human nose harbors a niche of olfactory ectomesenchymal stem cells displaying neurogenic and osteogenic properties. Stem Cells and Development. 2009;**19**(6):853-866

[222] Rui K, Zhang Z, Tian J, Lin X, Wang X, Ma J, et al. Olfactory ecto-mesenchymal stem cells possess immunoregulatory function and suppress autoimmune arthritis. Cellular & Molecular Immunology. 2016;**13**(3):401

[223] Ercolin ACM, Roballo KCS, Casals JB, Pieri NCG, Souza AF, Barreto RSN, et al. Rabbit olfactory stem cells. Isolation protocol and characterization. Acta Cirurgica Brasileira. 2016;**31**(1):59-66

[224] Altunbaş K, Yaprakci MV, Celik S. Isolation and characterization of olfactory stem cells from canine olfactory mucosa. Kafkas Universitesi Veteriner Fakultesi Dergisi. 2016;**22**(2):237-243. DOI: 10.9775/kvfd.2015.14277

[225] Veron AD, Bienboire-Frosini C, Feron F, Codecasa E, Deveze A, Royer D, et al. Isolation and characterization of olfactory ecto-mesenchymal stem cells from eight mammalian genera. BMC Veterinary Research. 2018;**14**(1):17

[226] Tomé M, Lindsay SL, Riddell JS, Barnett SC. Identification of nonepithelial multipotent cells in the embryonic olfactory mucosa. Stem Cells. 2009;**27**(9):2196-2208

[227] Johnstone SA, Liley M, Dalby MJ, Barnett SC. Comparison of human olfactory and skeletal MSCs using osteogenic nanotopography to demonstrate bone-specific bioactivity of the surfaces. Acta Biomaterialia. 2015;**13**:266-276

[228] Lindsay SL, Johnstone SA, Mountford JC, Sheikh S, Allan DB, Clark L, et al. Human mesenchymal stem cells isolated from olfactory biopsies but not bone enhance CNS myelination in vitro. Glia. 2013;**61**(3):368-382

[229] Shafiee A, Kabiri M, Ahmadbeigi N, Yazdani SO, Mojtahed M, Amanpour S, et al. Nasal septum-derived multipotent progenitors: A potent source for stem cell-based regenerative medicine. Stem Cells and Development. 2011;**20**(12):2077-2091

[230] King NM, Perrin J. Ethical issues in stem cell research and therapy. Stem Cell Research & Therapy. 2014;**5**(4):85

[231] Marshall CT, Guo Z, Lu C, Klueber KM, Khalyfa A, Cooper NG, et al. Human adult olfactory neuroepithelial derived progenitors retain telomerase activity and lack apoptotic activity. Brain Research. 2005;**1045**(1-2):45-56

[232] Antonevich N, Hancharou A, Buschik O, Rydna A, Chekan V, Strinkevich E, et al. Human olfactory mucosa-derived mesenchymal stem cells suppress cytotoxic functions of CD8+ T-lymphocytes and natural killer cells. Journal of Allergy and Clinical Immunology. 2018;**141**(2):AB122

[233] Steinbach S, Proft F, Schulze-Koops H, Hundt W, Heinrich P, Schulz S, et al. Gustatory and olfactory function in rheumatoid arthritis. Scandinavian Journal of Rheumatology. 2011;**40**(3):169-177

[234] McDonald C, Mackay-Sim A, Crane D, Murrell W. Could cells from your nose fix your heart? Transplantation of olfactory stem cells in a rat model of

cardiac infarction. The Scientific World Journal. 2010;**10**:422-433

[235] Murrell W, Wetzig A, Donnellan M, Féron F, Burne T, Meedeniya A, et al. Olfactory mucosa is a potential source for autologous stem cell therapy for Parkinson's disease. Stem Cells. 2008;**26**(8):2183-2192

[236] Veron AD, Bienboire-Frosini C, Girard SD, Sadelli K, Stamegna J-C, Khrestchatisky M, et al. Syngeneic transplantation of olfactory ectomesenchymal stem cells restores learning and memory abilities in a rat model of global cerebral ischemia. Stem Cells International. 2018;**2018**:1-10. DOI: 10.1155/2018/2683969

[237] Nivet E, Vignes M, Girard SD, Pierrisnard C, Baril N, Devèze A, et al. Engraftment of human nasal olfactory stem cells restores neuroplasticity in mice with hippocampal lesions. The Journal of Clinical Investigation. 2011;**121**(7):2808-2820

[238] Bas E, Van De Water TR, Lumbreras V, Rajguru S, Goss G, Hare JM, et al. Adult human nasal mesenchymal-like stem cells restore cochlear spiral ganglion neurons after experimental lesion. Stem Cells and Development. 2013;**23**(5):502-514

[239] Pandit SR, Sullivan JM, Egger V, Borecki AA, Oleskevich S. Functional effects of adult human olfactory stem cells on early-onset sensorineural hearing loss. Stem Cells. 2011;**29**(4):670-677

[240] Young E, Westerberg B, Yanai A, Gregory-Evans K. The olfactory mucosa: A potential source of stem cells for hearing regeneration. Regenerative Medicine. 2018;**13**(05):581-593. DOI: 10.2217/rme-2018-0009

[241] Toft A, Tomé M, Lindsay SL, Barnett SC, Riddell JS. Transplant-mediated repair properties of rat olfactory mucosal OM-I and OM-II sphere-forming cells. Journal of Neuroscience Research. 2012;**90**(3):619-631

[242] Xiao M, Klueber KM, Lu C, Guo Z, Marshall CT, Wang H, et al. Human adult olfactory neural progenitors rescue axotomized rodent rubrospinal neurons and promote functional recovery. Experimental Neurology. 2005;**194**(1):12-30

[243] Roche P, Alekseeva T, Widaa A, Ryan A, Matsiko A, Walsh M, et al. Olfactory derived stem cells delivered in a biphasic conduit promote peripheral nerve repair in vivo. Stem Cells Translational Medicine. 2017;**6**(10):1894-1904

[244] Kaplan HM, Mishra P, Kohn J. The overwhelming use of rat models in nerve regeneration research may compromise designs of nerve guidance conduits for humans. Journal of Materials Science: Materials in Medicine. 2015;**26**(8):226

[245] Tos P, Ronchi G, Papalia I, Sallen V, Legagneux J, Geuna S, et al. Methods and protocols in peripheral nerve regeneration experimental research: Part I—Experimental models. International Review of Neurobiology. 2009;**87**:47-79

[246] Pavić R, Pavić ML, Tvrdeić A, Tot OK, Heffer M. Rat sciatic nerve crush injury and recovery tracked by plantar test and immunohistochemistry analysis. Collegium Antropologicum. 2011;**35**(1):93-100

[247] Nichols CM, Myckatyn TM, Rickman SR, Fox IK, Hadlock T, Mackinnon SE. Choosing the correct functional assay: A comprehensive assessment of functional tests in the rat. Behavioural Brain Research. 2005;**163**(2):143-158

[248] Ozturk C. Peripheral nerve surgery models sciatic nerve crush injury model.

In: Plastic and Reconstructive Surgery. London: Springer-Verlag; 2015. pp. 513-517. DOI: 10.1007/978-1-4471-6335-0_63

[249] Dellon A, Mackinnon S. Sciatic nerve regeneration in the rat. Validity of walking track assessment in the presence of chronic contractures. Microsurgery. 1989;**10**(3):220-225

[250] Hayashi A, Moradzadeh A, Hunter DA, Kawamura DH, Puppala VK, Tung TH, et al. Retrograde labeling in peripheral nerve research: It is not all black and white. Journal of Reconstructive Microsurgery. 2007;**23**(07):381-389

[251] Carriel V, Garzón I, Alaminos M, Cornelissen M. Histological assessment in peripheral nerve tissue engineering. Neural Regeneration Research. 2014;**9**(18):1657

[252] Navarro X, Udina E. Methods and protocols in peripheral nerve regeneration experimental research: Part III—Electrophysiological evaluation. International Review of Neurobiology. 2009;**87**:105-126

[253] Zeidenberg J, Burks SS, Jose J, Subhawong TK, Levi AD. The utility of ultrasound in the assessment of traumatic peripheral nerve lesions: Report of 4 cases. Neurosurgical Focus. 2015;**39**(3):E3

[254] Shen N, Zhu J. Application of sciatic functional index in nerve functional assessment. Microsurgery. 1995;**16**(8):552-555

[255] de Medinaceli L, Freed WJ, Wyatt RJ. An index of the functional condition of rat sciatic nerve based on measurements made from walking tracks. Experimental Neurology. 1982;**77**(3):634-643

[256] Algora J, Chen LE, Seaber AV, Wong GH, Urbaniak JR. Functional effects of lymphotoxin on crushed peripheral nerve. Microsurgery: Official Journal of the International Microsurgical Society and the European Federation of Societies for Microsurgery. 1996;**17**(3):131-135

[257] Varejão AS, Cabrita AM, Meek MF, Bulas-Cruz J, Melo-Pinto P, Raimondo S, et al. Functional and morphological assessment of a standardized rat sciatic nerve crush injury with a non-serrated clamp. Journal of Neurotrauma. 2004;**21**(11):1652-1670

[258] Dinh P, Hazel A, Palispis W, Suryadevara S, Gupta R. Functional assessment after sciatic nerve injury in a rat model. Microsurgery: Official Journal of the International Microsurgical Society and the European Federation of Societies for Microsurgery. 2009;**29**(8):644-649

[259] Bain J, Mackinnon S, Hunter D. Functional evaluation of complete sciatic, peroneal, and posterior tibial nerve lesions in the rat. Plastic and Reconstructive Surgery. 1989;**83**(1):129-138

[260] Thalhammer J, Vladimirova M, Bershadsky B, Strichartz G. Neurologic evaluation of the rat during sciatic nerve block with lidocaine. The Journal of the American Society of Anesthesiologists. 1995;**82**(4):1013-1025

[261] Koka R, Hadlock TA. Quantification of functional recovery following rat sciatic nerve transection. Experimental Neurology. 2001;**168**(1):192-195

[262] Wong K-H, Kanagasabapathy G, Bakar R, Phan C-W, Sabaratnam V. Restoration of sensory dysfunction following peripheral nerve injury by the polysaccharide from culinary and medicinal mushroom, Hericium erinaceus (Bull.: Fr.) Pers. through its neuroregenerative action. Food Science and Technology. 2015;**35**(4):712-721

[263] Boissé L, Spencer SJ, Mouihate A, Vergnolle N, Pittman QJ. Neonatal immune challenge alters nociception in the adult rat. Pain. 2005;**119**(1-3):133-141

[264] Hu D, Hu R, Berde CB. Neurologic evaluation of infant and adult rats before and after sciatic nerve blockade. Anesthesiology: The Journal of the American Society of Anesthesiologists. 1997;**86**(4):957-965

[265] Bozkurt A, Tholl S, Wehner S, Tank J, Cortese M, Mon O'Dey D, et al. Evaluation of functional nerve recovery with Visual-SSI—A novel computerized approach for the assessment of the static sciatic index (SSI). Journal of Neuroscience Methods. 2008;**170**(1):117-122

[266] Varejão AS, Cabrita AM, Meek MF, Bulas-Cruz J, Filipe VM, Gabriel RC, et al. Ankle kinematics to evaluate functional recovery in crushed rat sciatic nerve. Muscle & Nerve: Official Journal of the American Association of Electrodiagnostic Medicine. 2003;**27**(6):706-714

[267] Maurício AC, Gärtner A, Armada-da-Silva P, Amado S, Pereira T, Veloso ANP, et al. Cellular systems and biomaterials for nerve regeneration in neurotmesis injuries. In: Biomaterials Applications for Nanomedicine. London: Intechopen; 2011. pp. 415-440. DOI: 10.5772/24247

[268] Raimondo S, Fornaro M, Di Scipio F, Ronchi G, Giacobini-Robecchi MG, Geuna S. Methods and protocols in peripheral nerve regeneration experimental research: Part II—Morphological techniques. International Review of Neurobiology. 2009;**87**:81-103

[269] Bozkurt A, Lassner F, O'Dey D, Deumens R, Böcker A, Schwendt T, et al. The role of microstructured and interconnected pore channels in a collagen-based nerve guide on axonal regeneration in peripheral nerves. Biomaterials. 2012;**33**(5):1363-1375

[270] Hirano A. The role of electron microscopy in neuropathology. Acta Neuropathologica. 2005;**109**(1):115-123

[271] Ronchi G, Jager SB, Vaegter CB, Raimondo S, Giacobini-Robecchi MG, Geuna S. Discrepancies in quantitative assessment of normal and regenerated peripheral nerve fibers between light and electron microscopy. Journal of the Peripheral Nervous System. 2014;**19**(3):224-233

Chapter 7

Risk and Reward: Avoiding Donor Morbidity and Maximizing Results in Nerve Transfer Surgery

Scott Ferris

Abstract

Nerve transfers have revolutionized outcomes in brachial plexus and peripheral nerve surgery. The ability to plan and execute effective and safe nerve transfers is now integral to providing contemporary reconstructive nerve surgery. This chapter provides an academic and philosophical approach to patient care. It includes details of preoperative planning and intraoperative techniques in sufficient practical detail to help surgeons both minimize risk and maximize results. This includes thorough discussion of techniques for interfasicular dissection, management of nerve branching, intraoperative nerve mapping, optimizing purity and quality of selected donor nerves and decision-making about donor neurotomy and preferred level of secondary nerve coaptation. These concepts and techniques provide the opportunity to improve results in known and familiar nerve transfers, as well as provide the opportunity to undertake new procedures with the best chance of success and the lowest risk of harm.

Keywords: nerve transfer, nerve injury, brachial plexus, peripheral nerve

1. Background

Nerve transfer surgery has revolutionized outcomes in both peripheral nerve and brachial plexus injuries. Despite first being described many decades ago, nerve transfers have not been widely adopted until recently [1, 2]. In essence, nerve transfers are attempts to repurpose existing functions toward more important, yet deficient functions. They require a full understanding of the deficit, and an ability to balance reconstructive needs with any potential donor sacrifice. This chapter aims to discuss donor morbidity in detail, which in almost all nerve surgery can be completely avoided with meticulous planning and technical care. By harvesting maximal donor nerve while avoiding donor morbidity, results with nerve transfer surgery can be safely optimized. It is incumbent upon all nerve surgeons to offer their patients the best possible result and the appropriate and sophisticated adoption and execution of nerve transfers will certainly contribute greatly to this cause.

2. An academic and philosophical approach to nerve transfer

The virtues of nerve transfer techniques are multiple. It is well accepted that one feature of nerve transfer surgery which portends an improved prognosis compared

IntechOpen

to grafting is that of the single neural coaptation [3]. Each neural coaptation has an obligate axonal dropout and therefore the fewer the coaptations the greater the number of axons which arrive at the end target irrespective of the original donor axon supply. It is additionally well known that by peripheral nerve transfers the surgeon is able to select deliberately either a pure or near pure motor or sensory axon pool for a motor or sensory reconstruction respectively. In the case of lower motor neuron injury, the surgeon is able to confirm the integrity of motor donor peripheral axons prior to using them for the reconstruction. A further advantage of nerve transfers when undertaken in the periphery for a peripheral target reconstruction is the short regeneration distance required [4]. There are many advantages of a short regeneration distance which all relate to time. The shorter the regeneration distance the earlier that the target receives its axonal input and therefore the less target organ attrition. In the case of motor reconstruction this means less motor endplate drop out. This enhances the number of motor fibers which can be recruited in the muscle and thereby enhances the amount of power which can be generated by the reanimated muscle. The shorter time between surgery and target reinnervation also means that surgery is still a reasonable proposition even if a patient has been referred late or has a delay to surgery for whatever reason. This therefore means that a greater pool of people can be assisted by virtue of this type of surgery compared to more traditional techniques.

Less discussed in the literature is the fact that many traditional reconstructions rely on a mixed motor and sensory donor nerve being utilized via a graft requiring two coaptations, in order to reconstruct a mixed motor and sensory recipient. This has a potentially profoundly negative impact of likelihood of reconstructive success. For illustration, if one accepts that each coaptation is associated with an approximate 50% axonal dropout then significant attrition occurs between the proximal donor and its distal targets. Assuming a 100% axon count in the reconstructive donor nerve the most axons that can arrive at the target is 25% having crossed two coaptations. If however one additionally considers a mixed 50% motor and 50% sensory donor is being used to reconstruct a mixed motor sensory recipient then this final target axon count is in fact 12.5%.

It is important to understand the reality that many traditional nerve grafting techniques are inherently unpredictable and imprecise reconstructive technique. The surgeon is then free to analyze individual clinical problems and attempt reconstructions based on techniques which both scientifically and experientially have a greater chance of success (**Table 1**).

	Nerve graft	**Nerve transfer**
Distance to target	Often long	Generally short
Number of coaptations	2	1
Donor axons	Often mixed motor/sensory	Usually specific
Quality of donor axons	Variable	Usually excellent by design
Early reinnervation	Sometimes	Usually
Suitable for late surgery	Uncommonly	Often
Operative scars and dissection	Long/multiple	Generally short and few

Table 1.
Comparison of nerve grafts and nerve transfers for reinnervation.

3. Intraoperative techniques

3.1 In transfers requiring intraneural neurolyses

The topography within peripheral nerves is extensively examined and discussed in the literature. It is often stated that this topography is critical to nerve transfer surgery in terms of selecting donor fascicles. While it is true that an understanding of this internal neural topography can expedite surgery and shorten operative times, reliance on internal topography at the expense of extensive intraneural dissection is in fact a risk for donor morbidity in nerve transfer surgery. The topography within an individual peripheral nerve although commonly similar between individuals is not uniform and as such the best way to minimize the risk of a donor deficit after harvesting a nerve for a nerve transfer, is an exhaustive and meticulous intraneural neurolysis and selective micro stimulation of individual fascicles and sub fascicles prior to a neurotomy.

In a transfer such as an ulnar fascicle to a nerve to biceps [5], it is this author's preferred technique to dissect the recipient nerve first. Once the likely site of nerve repair is known and allowing for the length that will be lost in transferring the donor fascicle to the recipient nerve, the site for exploration of the donor nerve is chosen. This sequence avoids unnecessarily dissecting donor nerves over a longer length than required, thereby reducing both operative time and inadvertent donor morbidity. At the chosen site and over a length of approximately 20 mm the ulnar nerve is dissected under the operating microscope by gently and bluntly teasing apart of individual fascicles. No division of axons is required to undertake this process. Each individual fascicle is looped with a small piece of background or colored vessel loop. Each piece of surgical background/vessel loop is clipped with a small or large crushing Weck clip which does not touch the nerve itself. These clips can be applied in a single, double, triple or quadruple fashion in order to label fascicles. In this way, it is easy to separately identify eight or more fascicles within a donor nerve (see **Figure 1**).

A chart can be constructed with these individual fascicles on the Y-axis and the observed function of these fascicles utilizing micro nerve stimulation on the X-axis. By separating these fascicles and insulating them from the other fascicles using dry microsurgical strolls, it is possible to see the distal function in the forearm or hand of each individual fascicle and document this in the chart (see **Figure 2**).

It is the author's preference to in fact undertake this stimulation at least twice for each fascicle, preferably separated by a time interval. Usually all fascicles are stimulated in turn and the chart is constructed. The chart is then observed to determine

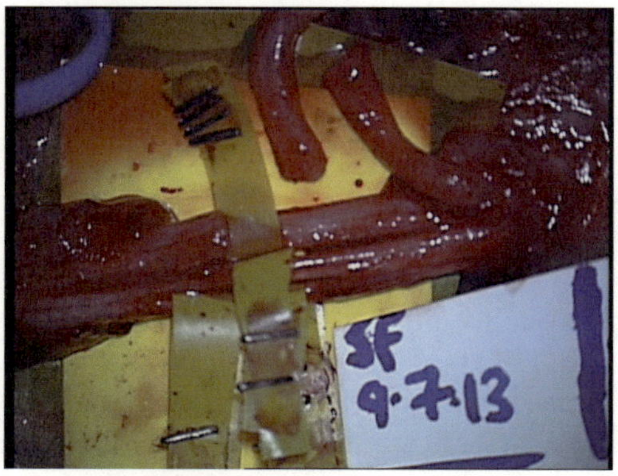

Figure 1.
Dissected and labeled ulnar nerve fascicles after neurotomy for secondary nerve repair to biceps nerve.

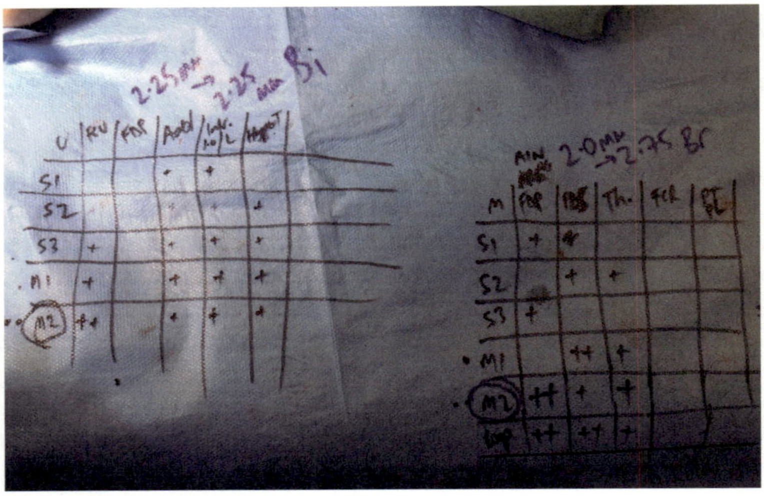

Figure 2.
Fascicular mapping chart. Note: "Y axis" with different fascicles listed and labeled, and "X axis" with intraoperative stimulation findings of those fascicles, and ultimate donors chosen circled and size matches listed on top to biceps (Bi) and brachialis (Br).

which fascicle or fascicles are most appropriate to be sacrificed for the nerve transfer. After this provisional decision has been made all fascicles are again stimulated. This is to ensure that the observed peripheral function remains the same and that no significant errors in stimulation, insulation, observation or recording have been made.

Given that the proposed donor nerve has now been observed to be functioning and its condition already evaluated without division under the operating microscope, the next step is to divide the recipient nerve. This division is undertaken as close to the biceps muscle as is possible to allow a tension free high quality nerve coaptation. Only now that the recipient nerve is observed to be in good condition for receipt of the nerve transfer at this level is the donor nerve sacrificed for use. The neurotomised fascicle(s) are then transferred and secondary nerve coaptation to the biceps nerve is undertaken under the operating microscope.

The technique described here for the ulnar to biceps nerve transfer can be utilized for any nerve transfer where the donor fascicle or nerve being used is less than the whole of the donor nerve being dissected. Other examples in common use are the partial median to brachialis and the partial contralateral C7 use for complete brachial plexus palsy. The same steps in the same order will maximize the surgeon's ability to provide maximal axonal input to the reconstruction while minimizing the risk of donor morbidity.

3.2 For nerve transfers not requiring intraneural neurolysis

In nerve transfers where no intraneural neurolysis is required to determine which axons will be used for the reconstruction, several of the previously discussed principles still apply. A good example of this is the triceps nerve(s) to the axillary nerve transfer [6]. It is usual for there to be approximately eight or so motor nerves to the triceps in the author's experience. It is important prior to deciding which nerve or nerves will be used in the reconstruction to determine each intact nerve to triceps' contribution to that triceps' function. Specifically the surgeon should observe each nerves diameter, length and the strength of contraction it elicits in the triceps when stimulated. The authors preferred stimulation is using a disposable nerve stimulator on its lowest setting of 0.5 mA. In this nerve transfer example one is therefore able sacrifice sufficient branches to triceps to maximize the axonal input

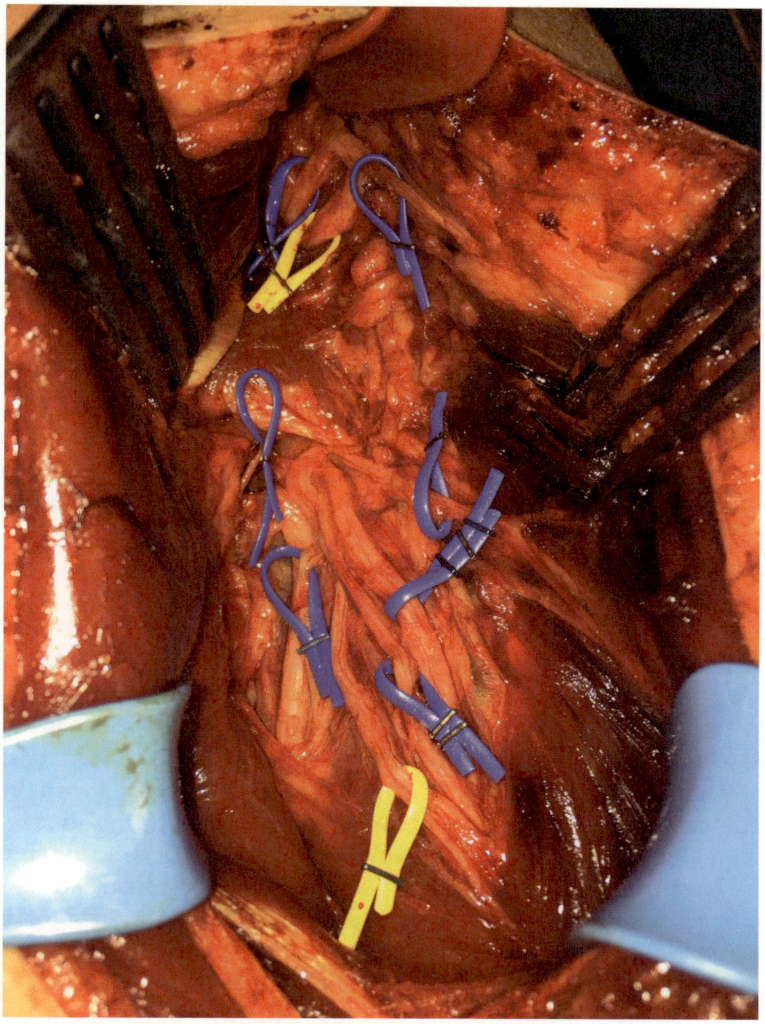

Figure 3.
Dissected and labeled triceps to axillary nerves. Note: Planned recipient anterior axillary nerve and donor triceps nerves looped in yellow ready for use; sensory posterior axillary nerve, dissected other triceps nerves plus radial nerve proper all looped in blue.

to the axillary nerve being reconstructed while maintaining sufficient function in the residual triceps. It would be an error to take a single branch triceps in a patient where multiple branches could safely be harvested because the axonal input for the reconstruction would therefore be less. Similarly it would be an error in these patients to take multiple branches of triceps without ensuring that there were multiple residual branches to maintain triceps function. Both of these potential errors can only be avoided by an exhaustive search for all nerves entering triceps and selectively isolating each and stimulating it to determine its function (**Figure 3**).

4. Decision-making about donor dissection, neurotomy level and branch management

Throughout the dissection of potential donor nerves, especially long nerves with multiple branches, it is important to be aware of the implications of the management of nerve branches, as well as the ultimate level for the donor neurotomy.

As one dissects any potential donor nerve, the more distal the ultimate neurotomy, the greater the preservation of proximal function can be, but the lower the axon count being used for the reconstruction. Also with a distal neurotomy and therefore long donor nerve, the nerve coaptation is closer to the target and benefits from a short regeneration distance as well as being more likely to be below the level of the nerve lesion. Alternatively, the more proximal the ultimate donor neurotomy, the greater the axon count being used for the reconstruction, but the greater the donor morbidity as well as increasing the regeneration distance and the risk of not being below the level of nerve injury (**Figure 4**).

An excellent example of this is when dissecting the mid and distal accessory nerve, commonly used for reanimation of the suprascapular nerve. In this situation the surgical goal is restoration of shoulder function, by reanimation of the supraspinatus and infraspinatus muscles. It is important to remember however, that the trapezius muscle also contributes to shoulder function. As such, there is a delicate balance between preserving maximal function in the upper trapezius muscle, while sacrificing and utilizing sufficient axons from lower trapezius (distal accessory nerve) for the reconstruction.

Performing the distal spinal accessory to suprascapular nerve transfer from a posterior approach facilitates management of the above issues. While the posterior approach requires lateral positioning of the patient and a more difficult dissection compared to an anterior approach, with care it allows full delineation of the donor and recipient anatomy before committing to any neurotomies. Once the recipient nerve has been dissected and evaluated, a decision can be made regarding what level on the SSN proper, or even the supraspinatus and infraspinatus nerves individually, the coaptation is planned. This level can be compared with the position, length, caliber, branching and potential pivot point of the mid-distal accessory nerve. It is desirable whenever possible, to preserve those branches into upper and middle trapezius which are too short to be used in the reconstruction, such that this component of trapezius is not denervated without any reconstructive benefit. Sometimes once all the exploratory surgical findings are known, if the suprascapular nerve approaching the notch is in excellent condition, then a decision can be made to use a slightly longer recipient nerve and a slightly shorter donor nerve

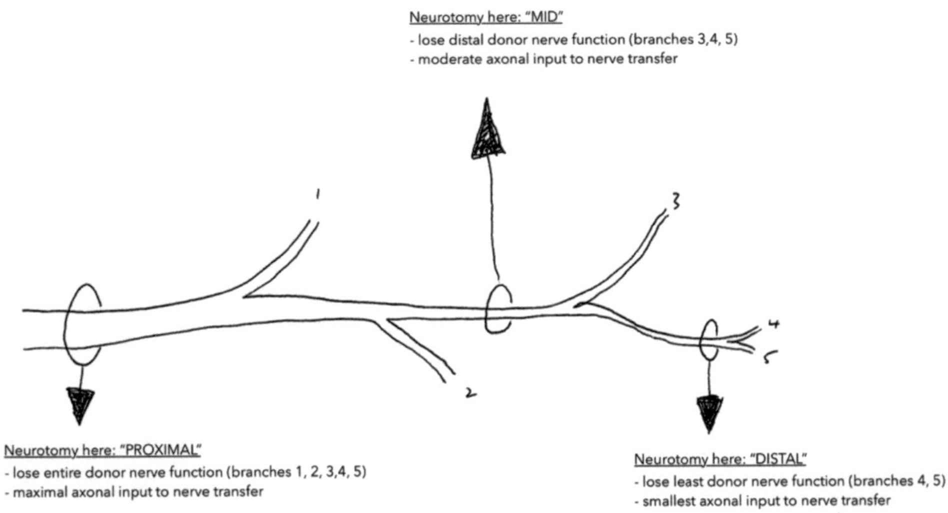

Figure 4.
Schematic representation of levels of donor neurotomy.

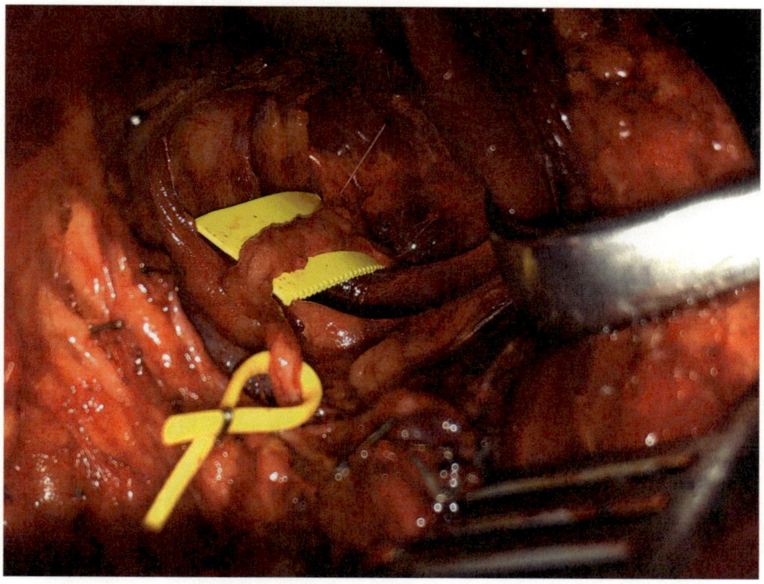

Figure 5.
Distal accessory nerve donor dissected. Note: Long length of donor dissected without needing to divide branches, and terminal branches diverging distally.

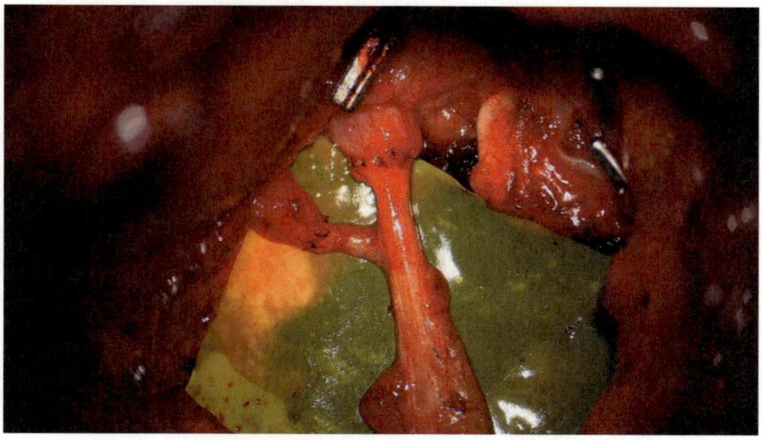

Figure 6.
Completed nerve repairs terminal accessory to both supraspinatus and infraspinatus nerves. Note: Posterior approach has allowed very distal repairs, close to target with good size matching, immediately distal to level of divided suprascapular ligament.

or lower pivot point in order to preserve the proximal and mid trapezius muscle branches. Only if such a trapezius branch still impedes tension free nerve transfer should it be sacrificed to prevent possible avulsion of the ultimate nerve repair (**Figures** 5 and **6**).

5. Optimizing purity and quality of donor nerves

It is important in all motor nerve transfers to keep motor donors as purely motor as possible in order to maximize target outcome as well as minimize sensory donor morbidity. When dissecting motor donor nerves for use, it is critical that where possible any sensory components or branches are identified such that they are not

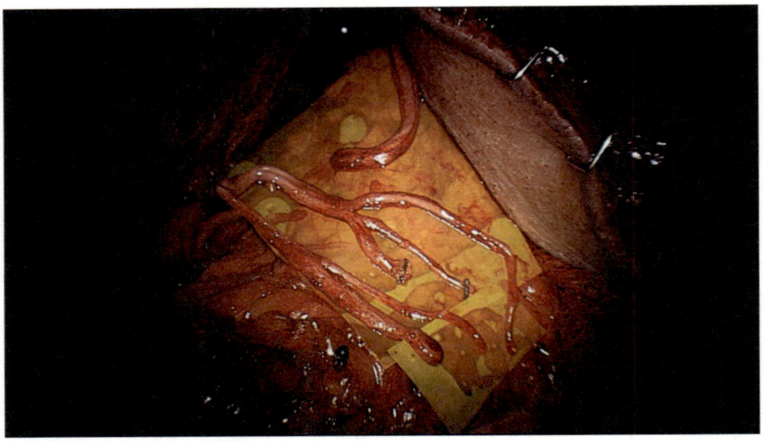

Figure 7.
Dissected and labeled intercostal nerves for gracilis flap. Note: Known sensory components of intercostal nerves labeled by small clips, with motor branches left unclipped ready to use to innervate free gracilis muscle flap, uppermost in picture.

inadvertently included in the nerve coaptation. Depending on the nature of the nerve transfer, techniques for this differ.

For fascicular nerve transfers, the insulated stimulation and selective fascicular mapping described above contributes greatly to this process. For triceps nerve donors the individual anatomical exploration and labeling of separate nerves achieves the same outcome of knowing which nerves are motor and adequately powered. One should always remember however that a fascicle or nerve which does not stimulate can either be a sensory fascicle, a temporarily neuropraxed fascicle, or a fascicle which has either a proximal or a distal permanent injury.

Intercostal nerve dissection is different due to the large sensory nerves which branch at intervals from what are mixed motor/sensory parent nerves. In these dissections, as one dissects along the intercostal nerve and finds what are clearly sensory branches, it is wise to use a small surgical clip applied to the end of these sensory nerves before they are divided, such that at a later stage they are clearly identifiable and used only for sensory targets. In this way the proportion of total axons which are actually motor axons ultimately used for motor reconstruction can be maximized.

The same techniques apply in reverse when dissecting sensory nerve donors, in order to not inadvertently include motor fibers in the reconstruction (**Figure** 7).

6. Patient selection

The techniques described here are very effective in restoring function when used in appropriate patients. Accurately determining which patients require which operations at what time point is the first step toward success.

Patients must have a stable skeleton with supple joints. They must also be available, motivated and cognitively capable of undergoing their postoperative rehabilitation.

The timing of surgery is critical. For a known open nerve lesion, reconstruction is best undertaken as soon as there is an appropriately skilled team and resourced operating theater. By contrast, the common closed avulsion lesions generally require greater investigation and preoperative assessment to determine whether surgery is necessary, or whether spontaneous recovery is likely. In this way, unnecessary surgery on spontaneously reversible neuropraxic lesions can be avoided.

In all acute or subacute patients, once it is clear that nerve reconstruction will be required, surgery should be scheduled as soon as possible such that the denervation time of native muscles requiring reinnervation is minimized.

In patients referred very late, there can paradoxically be less urgency. This is because in these patients there is no meaningful chance of reinnervating their native muscles. In these patients, active function is achieved by either pedicled transfer of intact regional muscle/tendon units, or by importing a free functioning muscle flap. In both pedicled or free muscle transfer it is possible to take the time to optimize the passive range of motion of all joints, as well as undertake preeducation and training of the patient before their definitive surgery because the urgency of reinnervating their original muscles is not present in such cases. In the case of pedicled muscle/tendon transfer there is no denervation time because no neurotomy and nerve repair is required. In the case of a free functioning muscle flap, the denervation time begins at the time of reconstruction, rather than at the time of initial injury, as the transferred free muscle flap is neurotized by using nerve transfer.

7. Example cases

7.1 Case 1: complete musculocutaneous nerve palsy as part of C56 palsy

A 32-year-old man sustained complete left C56 root avulsions in a motorbike accident. Four months later he underwent multiple reconstructions by nerve transfer, including median to brachialis and ulnar to biceps nerve transfers. By 15 months postoperatively, he could flex his elbow with at least 12 kg dumbbell in his hand (**Figure 8**).

7.2 Case 2: failed axillary nerve grafting—salvage with triceps nerve transfer

A 17-year-old footballer while undergoing a right shoulder stabilization procedure sustained an iatrogenic combined nerve and arterial injury. He had immediate

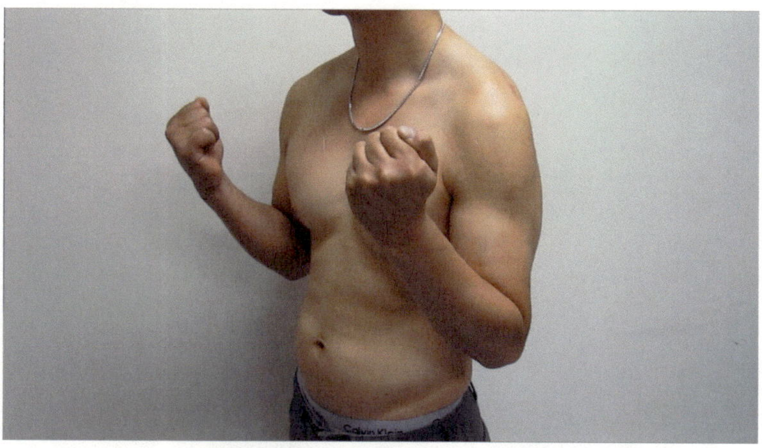

Figure 8.
Postoperative result of nerve transfers to biceps and brachialis. Note: Excellent restoration of muscle bulk and range of elbow flexion.

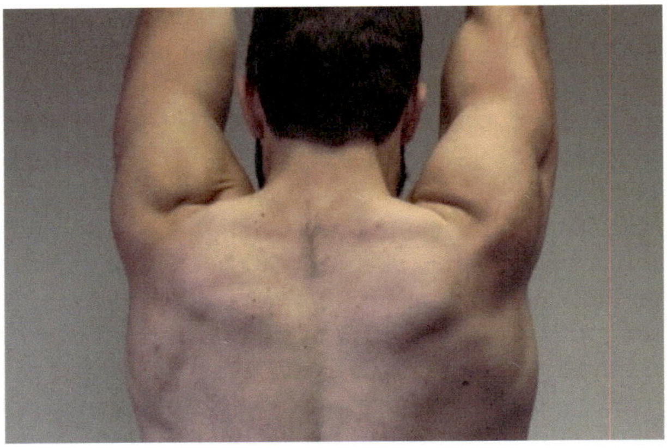

Figure 9.
Postoperative result of salvage nerve transfer using triceps donors to right axillary nerve. Note: Full abduction of shoulder, with excellent bulk of deltoid.

vascular repair, and axillary nerve grafting on day four after injury. When at 8 months after grafting there was no evidence of nerve regeneration or muscle reinnervation, he was taken back for exploration and underwent a salvage nerve transfer using two separate triceps nerves to reanimate the extreme distal end of the anterior branch of his axillary nerve (**Figure 9**).

7.3 Case 3: complete brachial plexus palsy-free muscle flap with accessory nerve transfer

A 39-year-old man was referred with a complete right brachial plexus palsy after a motorbike accident into a tree. He underwent multiple reconstructions, including a free functioning gracilis muscle flap, innervated by the spinal accessory nerve transfer, which was undertaken 5 months after his injury. This muscle was inset proximally on the clavicle and tunneled distally in the arm, under a PT/FCR pulley at the elbow, to all four FDP tendons, thereby acting as both and elbow flexor and a finger flexor (**Figure 10**).

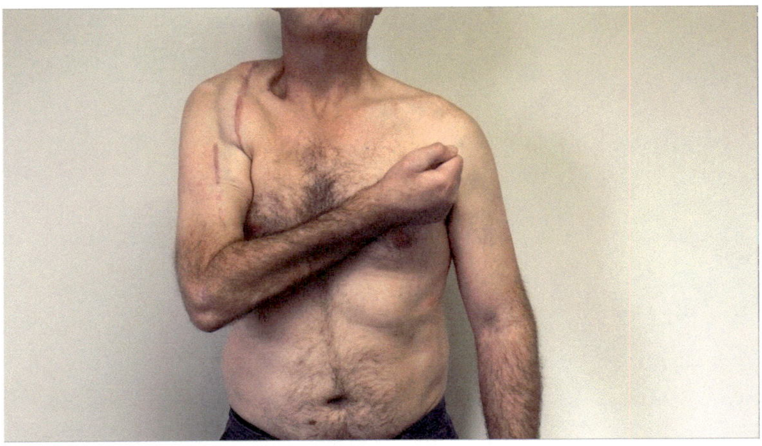

Figure 10.
Postoperative result of free functioning gracilis muscle, innervated by accessory nerve transfer. Note: Bulk of reinnervated gracilis muscle superiorly and excellent active range of elbow flexion restored.

8. Conclusions

Nerve transfers have completely transformed the expected surgical outcomes for many nerve deficits and patterns of nerve injury. The way in which nerve transfers are used depends on individual patterns of and time since injury. The best possible outcomes depend on careful balancing of the risks and rewards in each individual patient. Informed, realistic and strategic preoperative planning, combined with meticulous intraoperative dissection, diligent appraisal of intraoperative findings and considered intraoperative decision-making prior to final execution of technically optimized nerve transfers allows the minimization of donor morbidity and maximization of surgical outcome.

Author details

Scott Ferris
Plastic and Reconstructive Surgeon, Australia

*Address all correspondence to: scott@scottferris.com.au

References

[1] Lurge A. On the use of n. musculocutaneous for neurotization on n. radialis in cases of very large defects of the latter. Annals of Surgery. 1948;**128**(1):110-115

[2] Nath RK, Mackinnon SE. Nerve transfers in the upper extremity. Hand Clinics. 2000;**16**(1):131-139, ix

[3] Mackinnon SE, Novak CB. Nerve transfers. New options for reconstruction following nerve injury. Hand Clinics. 1999;**15**(4):643-666, ix

[4] Tung TH, Mackinnon SE. Brachial plexus injuries. Clinics in Plastic Surgery. 2003;**30**(2):269-287

[5] Oberlin C, Béal D, Leechavengong S, Salon A, Dauge MC, Sarcy JJ. Nerve transfer to biceps muscle using part of ulnar nerve for C5-C6 avulsion of the brachial plexus: Anatomical study and report of four cases. Journal of Hand Surgery (American Volume). 1994;**19**:232-237

[6] Leechavengvongs S, Witoonchart K, Uerpairojkit C, Thuvasethakul P. Nerve transfer to deltoid muscle using the nerve to the long head of the triceps, part II: A report of 7 cases. Journal of Hand Surgery. 2003;**28A**:633-638

Section 3

New Insights For Neuropathic Pain

Chapter 8

Peripheral Sensitization

Si-Qi Wei, Zhuo-Ying Tao, Yang Xue and Dong-Yuan Cao

Abstract

Peripheral sensitization indicates increased responsiveness and reduced threshold of nociceptive neurons in the periphery to the stimulation, which usually occurs after peripheral tissue injury and inflammation. As an integral part of pain, peripheral sensitization and its mechanisms have received much attention, and numerous types of neurotransmitters and chemicals related to peripheral sensitization were investigated. We developed an animal model of peripheral sensitization, and it provides evidence that some neurotransmitters, such as glutamate and substance P, release from adjacent peripheral nerves contributing to the peripheral sensitization of pathological pain. In this chapter, we reviewed the advances in peripheral sensitization, and it will provide a basis for new targets to attenuate pain of peripheral origin.

Keywords: pain, peripheral sensitization, tissue injury, inflammation, neurotransmitter, ion channel

1. Introduction

Peripheral sensitization refers to reduced threshold and augmented response of the sensory nerve fibers in the peripheral to external stimulus, which is manifested as enhanced stimulus-dependent pain called primary hyperalgesia [1]. Commonly, peripheral sensitization occurs following peripheral nerve injury, tissue injury, and inflammation. Tissue injury may accompany the injury of peripheral nerve endings to some content. The endogenous chemicals released from the site of tissue injury or inflammation can activate and sensitize the peripheral sensory neurons, resulting in peripheral sensitization [2, 3]. Similar sensitization phenomenon taking place in the central nervous system is called central sensitization, which may be initially induced by peripheral sensitization [4, 5]. The peripheral sensitization and central sensitization together produce neuropathic pain and inflammatory pain reflected as allodynia and hyperalgesia. However, there is no satisfactory therapy for the management of allodynia and hyperalgesia.

Peripheral sensitization increases the release of the neurotransmitters from the peripheral endings and the terminals of the spinal cord, aggravating the neurogenic inflammation and nociception. Pain usually starts with the activation of peripheral sensory neurons which subsequently process and convey nociceptive message to spinal cord and brain regions. That is, to some extent, the inhibition of peripheral sensitization may prevent the subsequent central events. For the pain management, local drug delivery can focus on the specific peripheral mechanisms including transduction and transmission of nociceptive signaling to limit both peripheral and central sensitization processes [6]. These facts increase the necessity to investigate the exclusive mechanisms of peripheral sensitization. Thus, in this chapter, we

IntechOpen

focus on the advances in peripheral sensitization, and it may contribute to the improvements of new therapies relieving pain of peripheral origin.

2. Peripheral nociceptors

Nociception is a process that different stimuli (thermal, mechanical, and chemical) are detected by the peripheral nerve fibers called nociceptor, through which the noxious stimuli are transduced into action potentials and conducted to the spinal cord and brain [7]. Unlike other sensory modalities that respond to innocuous stimulus such as touch, nociceptors are only activated by noxious stimuli that could be harmful to the organism. The nociceptor consists of three parts: the axon, cell body, and central terminals. The cell bodies of the nociceptors are located in the dorsal root ganglia (DRG) for the body and the trigeminal ganglia (TG) for the maxillofacial region, and they are always connected to the afferent fibers. The site where the terminals of the fibers respond to peripheral stimuli is known as the receptive field. According to the type of the afferent fibers, the nociceptor can be divided into myelinated Aδ fibers and unmyelinated C fibers. Many of the unmyelinated fibers respond to a wide range of noxious stimuli [8]. Nociceptors can send and receive the messages from both the central and peripheral terminals [5, 7]. Following injury and inflammation, the nociceptors may become sensitized by pro-nociceptive mediators, such as prostaglandins, bradykinin, substance P (SP), extracellular ATP, and protons [9]. The activation of the nociceptors is related to the site of the stimuli application and stimuli modality including chemical, thermal (hot and cold), and mechanical modalities [8]. Several changes in nociceptors may account for the peripheral sensitization. First, the thresholds of primary afferent Aδ and C fibers lower in response to innoxious stimuli. Second, Aδ and C fibers at the site of tissue injury or inflammation exhibit enhanced responses to supra-threshold mechanical or heat stimuli. Third, adjacent receptive fields of Aδ and C fibers increase innervation to the injured site [10].

3. Challenges in developing effective drugs

Although considerable progress has been made in investigating the role of peripheral sensitization in nociceptive processing during the past decades, pain researches bear burdens in translation from pre-clinical studies to successful clinical intervention. Several reasons may explain why the effective analgesics develop slowly. First, the complicated mechanisms of different patients in distinct pain states and the diversity types and functions of mediators in different pain pathways may be barriers in developing effective therapies [7, 11]. Second, currently available analgesic drugs targeting pain mechanisms produce serious side-effects and unsatisfactory efficacy [2, 11, 12]. As is known to all, the most popular analgesia drug, opioid, is hampered by desirable side-effects such as tolerance, respiratory depression, and addiction [13, 14]. The transient receptor potential vanilloid 1 (TRPV1) antagonists have side-effects such as loss of the noxious heat sensation, increased burn risk, and hyperthermia [15]. Obviously, these challenges drive us to find drugs targeting selectively on modulation of peripheral mechanisms and not crossing the blood-brain-barrier, through which the side-effects may be avoided. To reduce potential systemic side-effects and improve compliance, there is a growing interest in "targeted peripheral analgesics" for further investigation and clinical use [6].

4. Animal model

Several animal models of various pain states have been established to investigate the mechanisms of peripheral sensitization, for example, inflammation pain models, neuropathic pain evoked by disease or damage to peripheral nerves, and post-operative pain models. Animal models of inflammatory pain have used a number of different irritants that are injected into skin, paw, muscle, joint, and visceral organ. Carrageenan, complete Freund's adjuvant (CFA), and capsaicin are commonly used inflammatory irritants to induce hyperalgesia. Common nerve injury models include: (1) ligating or transecting the spinal nerves, such as spinal nerve ligation model (SNL); (2) ligating or lesioning the sciatic nerve, such as chronic constriction injury (CCI); and (3) ligating distal branches (peroneal and tibial) of the sciatic nerve (spared nerve injury) [16].

To better understand the mechanisms of transmission between peripheral sensory nerve endings, we have successfully established an electrophysiological animal model in which antidromic electrical stimulation of a sensory nerve excites the adjacent primary afferents from the different spinal segments [17]. In this model, two adjacent cutaneous branches of spinal dorsal rami in the thoracic segments, T9 and T10, were dissociated and transected proximally from the spinal cord in anesthetized rats. Then antidromic electrical stimulation with 0.5 ms pulse duration, 20 Hz frequency, and 1 mA intensity was applied to T9 spinal nerve branch, and the nerve activities of T10 nerve branch were recorded [18]. All recorded afferent neurons from the T10 cutaneous branch were classified as Aβ, Aδ, and C fibers according to the conduction velocity and the receptive properties [19]. The discharges of the isolated Aβ, Aδ, and C fibers of the T10 cutaneous branch were significantly enhanced by antidromic electrical stimulation of the adjacent T9 spinal nerve branch [18]. It is in line with our previous studies that antidromic stimulation of T9 spinal nerve branch can activate and sensitize Aβ, Aδ, and C fibers obtained from the adjacent T10 dorsal cutaneous branch [20–23]. The activation and sensitization of these fibers not only occur between the peripheral sensory nerve terminals, but also conduct nociceptive impulses to the central nerve system [17, 24]. The increase in neural discharges of the peripheral fibers caused by the electrical stimulation of adjacent cutaneous nerves mimicked the effects of released chemicals at the peripheral nerve endings [25]. On the basis of this model, the effects of antidromic electrical stimulation of spinal cutaneous branches on the discharge activities of remote mechanoreceptive units were observed. It was found that antidromic stimulation of either T8 or T9 dorsal cutaneous branch significantly increased the discharge activities of the remote T12 nerve, and the increasing time after the electrical stimulation was delayed as the distance increased between the stimulated branch and the recorded one [26].

In these experiments, both nerve branches of the adjacent segments were isolated from the central nervous system; the activation of nerve fibers at one segment by antidromic electrical stimulation affects an adjacent segment suggesting that electrical and chemical signals are transmitted from the stimulated nerves to the recorded fibers without any involvement of the central nervous system. Electrical stimulation of the nerve directly induces the release of chemicals; these chemicals and substances through diffusion produce afferent impulses of adjacent nerve endings and also cause release of neurotransmitters at the adjacent peripheral nerve endings, a process known as axon reflex [17, 23, 26, 27].

5. Mechanisms of peripheral sensitization

There are two processes implicated in peripheral sensitization: (1) early post-translational changes in the peripheral terminals of nociceptors, for example, the

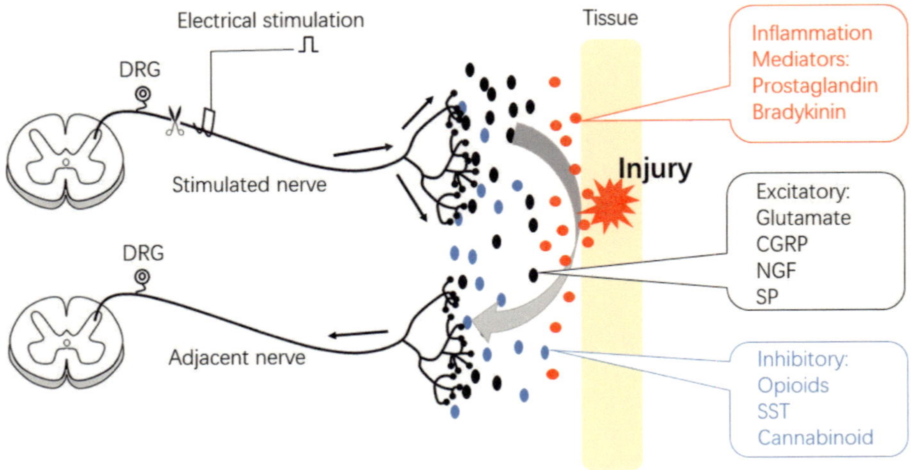

Figure 1.
After tissue injury, chemicals such as inflammatory mediators and neurotransmitters released from the injury site or the nerve endings activate the receptors and channels on the adjacent peripheral nerve terminals, subsequently resulting in peripheral sensitization. In our electrophysiological model, antidromic electrical stimulation of one nerve branch induces the release of neurotransmitters and modulators into the peripheral tissues to mimic tissue injury condition. The released chemicals diffuse to the adjacent peripheral nerve terminals and induce peripheral sensitization. Abbreviations: CGRP, calcitonin gene-related peptide; DRG, dorsal root ganglion; NGF, nerve growth factor; SP, substance P; SST, somatostatin.

phosphorylation of the ion channels prolongs depolarization and enhances response by lowering the open threshold or prolonging the open time of channels; (2) altered gene expression, changing transcription or translation of certain protein [10, 28]. For instance, deletion or silencing of calcitonin gene-related peptide alpha (αCGRP) gene expression drastically reduces TRPV1 potentiation in peptidergic nociceptors by abrogating its Ca^{2+}-dependent exocytotic recruitment [29].

Peripheral sensitization results from sensitization and excitation of the primary afferent neurons following tissue injury and inflammation. When a peripheral nerve is injured, the distal stump of injured axons undergoes Wallerian degeneration, i.e., breakdown of myelin sheaths, recruitment of inflammatory cells from the circulation, and over-production of growth factors and pro-inflammatory cytokines or mediators. These cytokines and mediators not only promote the regeneration of injured axons but also activate and sensitize nociceptors [30]. During the process of sensitization, the inflammation mediators either bind to different receptors or activate second messenger systems, resulting in the modification of the ion channels [31]. Primary targets of these mediators are ion channels; the activation of either the voltage-gated channel or the ligand-gated channel enhances the number of the action potentials, a process known as sensitization. A wide range of chemicals, such as nerve growth factors (NGF), bradykinin, SP, prostaglandins, opioids, and glutamate, contribute to the peripheral sensitization (**Figure 1**). The following section will address inflammatory mediators, ion channels, and neurotransmitter receptors involved in peripheral sensitization.

6. Inflammatory mediator

Bradykinin and prostaglandin have attracted much attention among inflammatory mediators. The inflammatory mediator prostaglandin E2, released from the inflamed tissue surrounding the terminals of sensory neurons or from endothelial cells after surgical trauma, contributes to the abnormal pain responses in inflammation pain and neuropathic pain. Peripheral injection of nonselective and selective cyclooxygenase (COX) inhibitors attenuates neuropathic pain following partial sciatic nerve transection [32], indicating that pro-inflammatory prostaglandins are involved in the development of neuropathic pain. Both morphological and pharmacological evidence indicate that peripheral prostaglandins are involved in the maintenance of neuropathic pain following nerve injury [30]. In a study using a thoracic muscle incision model to characterize post-operative pain-related behaviors, tissue prostaglandin E2 increased in surgery animals compared with the sham-operated control animals under the same anesthesia, indicating that prostaglandin E2 is associated with post-operative pain [33]. Prostaglandin also participated in the long-lasting sensitization of nociceptors in acute inflammation induced by carrageenan in mice [34].

Bradykinin is an important neuropeptide released after tissue injury. Upon release, bradykinin affects nociceptive afferents through activation of two pharmacologically distinctive receptors designated B2 and B1, respectively [35, 36]. An increased B1 receptor gene expression was found in peripheral neural tissue in CFA-induced mechanical hyperalgesia, and the selective bradykinin B1 receptor antagonist BI113823 reduced CFA-induced mechanical hyperalgesia [37]. Activation of bradykinin receptors promoted nociceptor sensitization and hyperalgesia by activating the protein kinase C (PKC) second-messenger system [38]. A study on CCI model showed that there was an increase in the mRNA expression of both B1 and B2 receptors in lumbar DRG following CCI. Furthermore, pharmacological antagonists of these receptors alleviate pain hypersensitivity associated with nerve injury [39]. Bradykinin-mediated sensitization of heat responses in C mechanoheat-sensitive fibers of isolated rat skin-saphenous nerve was significantly attenuated by the COX-1 and COX-2 inhibitors [40].

7. Ion channels

The electrical activity of primary afferent neurons is primarily governed by the expression and function of ion channels that define the resting membrane potential, action potential initiation, depolarization and repolarization, refractory period between action potentials, and transmitter release from their terminals in the dorsal horn. In this part, we will review the voltage-gated channel transient receptor potential vanilloid (TRPV), voltage-gated sodium channels, and voltage-gated calcium channels (VGCCs), which may be dysregulated underlying peripheral sensitization.

7.1 The voltage-gated channel transient receptor potential vanilloid

The TRPV is one of the subfamilies of the transient receptor potential (TRP) through which the external stimuli are transduced to electrical impulses. Based on amino acid sequence homology, members of this family in the mammalian have been classified into six subfamilies: TRPA (ankyrin), TRPV (vanilloid), TRPM (melastatin), TRPC (canonical), TRPP (polycystin), and TRPML (mucolipin) [41]. TRP channels are tetramers composed of identical subunits, which have six transmembrane domains and cytoplasmic amino and carboxy termini [42].

7.1.1 TRPV1

TRPV1 is a non-selective cation ion channel which is largely located in small-diameter neurons with C fiber axons [43] in DRG innervating body and TG innervating oral and maxillofacial regions. Similar to voltage-gated sodium channels, TRPV1 exhibits radial symmetry around a central ion channel which is formed by transmembrane segments 5–6 (S5–S6) and the intervening pore loop and is flanked by S1–S4 domains [42]. TRPV1 is a polymodal receptor which can be activated by a wide range of stimuli including capsaicin [44], other endogenous lipids, acidic pH [43], and noxious heat (>42°C) [44]. TRPV1 upregulation in sensory neurons is a key element in pain development and maintenance of several chronic pathological conditions. Recently, the abundance of the evidence suggests that the TRPV1 receptor is one of the key targets for developing new analgesics.

7.1.2 TRPV1 and pain

It is widely acknowledged that TRPV1 contributes to heat and mechanical sensitization. Injection of capsaicin into the skin in humans produces a burning sensation and flare response, the area of application becomes insensitive to mechanical and thermal stimulation, the area of flare exhibits a primary hyperalgesia to mechanical and thermal stimuli, and an area beyond the flare exhibits secondary allodynia [45, 46]. Through the activation of TRPV1 by the capsaicin and other pungent compounds, burning pain may be produced via depolarizing specific subsets of Aδ and C nociceptors [44]. The TRPV1 population is also required for the development of thermal and mechanical hyperalgesia after CFA injection [47, 48]. Knockout of TRPV1 or pretreatment with the TRPV1 antagonists, AMG9810 or 5′-iodoresiniferatoxin (5′-IRTX), significantly reduced complement C5a-induced mechanical sensitization, indicating that TRPV1 activity is required for maintaining C5a-induced mechanical hypersensitivity [49]. The TRPV1 can assess the physiological environment of the sensory nerve terminal and alter neuronal responsiveness in the context of tissue injury [43]. The mechanical allodynia and thermal hyperalgesia were alleviated in Pirt (a membrane protein which binds to TRPV1 to enhance its activity) knockout mice in CCI models, and the increase in TRPV1 expression was less in Pirt knockout mice in CCI models, suggesting that Pirt together with TRPV1 is involved in CCI-induced neuropathic pain [50].

7.1.3 Activation of the TRPV1

The activation of TRPV1 increases the calcium permeability of the receptor, priming membrane depolarization and subsequent sensory neuron activation [44, 51]. The TRPV1 receptor occupancy triggers Na^+ and Ca^{2+} influx, action potential firing, and the consequent burning sensation associated with spicy food or capsaicin-induced pain [44]. TRPV1 can be sensitized via the second messenger signaling cascade in response to various pro-inflammation mediators and chemicals like bradykinin, lipids, and prostaglandins [44]. A multitude of lipids modulate the TRP-channels through G-protein coupled receptor via different signaling pathways [52]. TRPV1 contributes to the persistence of remifentanil-induced both thermal and mechanical post-operative hyperalgesia through the trafficking of N-methyl-D-aspartate (NMDA) receptors via the activation of calmodulin-dependent protein kinase (CaMKII)-PKC but not protein kinase A (PKA) signaling pathways in DRG neurons [53]. Bradykinin sensitizes TRPV1 through enhancing the excitability of the peptidergic C-type nociceptor end and the neuronal exocytosis of large dense core vesicles containing αCGRP [54]. Tumor necrosis factor-α (TNF-α) can sensitize TRPV1 by promoting its expression, thus leading to mechanical allodynia and thermal hyperalgesia in vincristine-treated rats [55]. NGF causes a long-lasting sensitization of nociceptor endings, in particular to thermal and chemical stimuli, which can be attributed to up-regulated TRPV-1 receptors in sensory endings [56].

The phosphorylation of TRPV1 has been shown to cause sensitization of the channel. The first report of the co-expression pattern of two ligand-gated channels, TRPV1 and P2X3 in TG, demonstrating that pretreatment with αβ-meATP (a selective P2X3 agonist) results in phosphorylation and sensitization of TRPV1, thus contributes to the peripheral sensitization known to underlie masseter hyperalgesia [57]. Activation of the metabotropic glutamate receptor (mGluR) 1/5 leads to phosphorylation of a specific TRPV1 residue via PKC and A-kinase–anchoring protein (AKAP) 150 in trigeminal sensory neurons, and functional interactions between glutamate receptors and TRPV1 mediate mechanical hyperalgesia in the muscle tissue [58]. A recent study found that the temperature sensitivity of TRPV1 channels are enhanced by SUMOylation of TRPV1 protein at a C-terminal Lys residue, indicating that SUMOylation of TRPV1 is essential for the key mechanism underlying peripheral sensitization and the development of inflammatory thermal hyperalgesia [59].

7.1.4 Other TRP receptors

Sensory neurons also express other TRP receptors besides TRPV1. TRPA1 is initiated by noxious cold (17°C), natural oils such as cinnamaldehyde and mustard oil, and inflammatory mediators [60]. TRPA1 is demonstrated to be cold sensitive [61] and plays roles in both cold transduction and mechanotransduction in cutaneous sensory neurons. AKAP 79/150 facilitates phosphorylation and sensitization of TRPA1 in peripheral sensory neurons, resulting in persistent mechanical hypersensitivity [62]. Another study also indicated that TRPA1 activation could co-sensitize TRPV1 channels [60]. Similar to TRPV1, TRPM8 is temperature sensitive and partly expressed by the somatosensory neurons in the DRG and TG. TRPM8 is activated by cool/cold temperature starting in the innocuous range (18–23°C) and cooling compounds such as menthol and icilin [63]. TRPV3 and TRPV4 have also been cloned and are heat sensors. TRPV3 was found to be responsible for detecting innocuous warm temperature ranging from 31 to 39°C. TRPV3 knockout mice had strong deficit in response to innocuous heat sensitivity but not in other sensory modalities [64]. TRPV4, which is expressed in small or medium diameter neurons with overlap in expression with TRPV1 [65], is activated by phorbol ester, innocuous temperature with a threshold higher than 27°C, low pH, citrate, endocannabinoids, arachidonic acid metabolites, and nitric oxide (NO) [66]. The evidence showed that TRPV4 was implicated in the transduction of mechanical stimuli and the development of mechanical hyperalgesia [3].

7.2 The voltage-gated sodium channel

Voltage-gated sodium ion channels are integral membrane proteins comprising a pore-forming α-subunit and two accessory β-subunits [67]. To date, nine isoforms of α subunit voltage-gated sodium channel (Na_v1.1–1.9), which display various channel properties and selective tissue distribution, have been discovered. A variety of voltage-gated sodium channels are expressed in somatosensory neurons, including the tetrodotoxin-sensitive (TTX-S) channels Na_v1.1, 1.6 and 1.7 and the tetrodotoxin-resistant (TTX-R) channels Na_v1.8 and 1.9. Voltage-gated sodium channels are essential for the generation and conductance of action potentials and therefore a crucial factor in neuronal excitability. The functions of voltage-gated sodium ion channels are regulated by their expression level, channel properties, and subcellular distribution. If some drugs block sodium-channels, the conduction of action potentials will be prevented, for instance, the local anesthetics can be used to abolish pain due to blocking sodium channels. Acting as a broad acting sodium blocker, phenytoin may inhibit overactivities of small fibers and reduce pain in small fiber neuropathic pain and diabetic neuropathic pain [68].

7.2.1 Na_v1.7

Na_v1.7 is of high interest because it functions as a kind of non-opioid analgesics. Na_v1.7, encoded by a sodium channel voltage-gated IX alpha subunit gene (SCN9A), is highly enriched within DRG and TG peripheral sensory neurons, as well as sympathetic neurons and olfactory epithelia [67, 69]. In rodent, Na_v1.7 is expressed within the soma of small-diameter DRG neurons and along the peripheral and central C fibers from these cells [70]. However, it was found that human DRG had a high ratio of Na_v1.7 expression and low ratio of Na_v1.8 expression compared to mouse DRG, indicating that Na_v1.7 mRNA predominantly expressed voltage-gated sodium channels in human DRG tissue [71]. Expression of Na_v1.7 is also detected in the preterminal central branches and terminals in the dorsal horn, as well as at nodes of Ranvier in a subpopulation of small-diameter myelinated fibers [72].

7.2.2 Na_v1.7 and pain

Na_v1.7 serves a remarkable function in pain perception. The Na_v1.7 knockout animals lose acute noxious mechanical sensation and inflammatory pain [73]. Mice lacking Na_v1.7 in sensory neurons showed reduced hypersensitivity to selected neuropathic pain and inflammatory pain models [74]. It has been found that injection of carrageenan increases expression of Na_v1.3 and Na_v1.7 and TTX-S currents in DRG neurons [75]. Estradiol upregulates TG Na_v1.7 mRNA and protein expression, thus inducing sex-differences of nociception in temporomandibular disorders (TMD) and hyperalgesia of the inflamed temporomandibular joint (TMJ) [75]. Besides, Na_v1.7 may interact with other signaling systems, such as endogenous opioids which are upregulated in the absence of Na_v1.7 and thought to feedback onto DRG neurons and/or terminals to suppress their excitability [76]. The qPCR analysis revealed a significant and dose-dependent increase in Na_v1.7 mRNA expression after the treatment of paclitaxel, which is a widely used chemotherapeutic drug that induces neuropathy and neuropathic pain, and the transient Na^+ currents and action potential firing frequency in small-diameter human DRG neurons also increased [71].

7.2.3 SCN9A genes and Na_v1.7

Recently, the mechanisms underlying several human pain disorders have been identified to be related to inherited mutations in the sodium channel genes expressed in damage-sensing neurons. The Na_v1.7 is encoded by the SCN9A gene. Inherited primary erythromelalgia is resulted from mutations of the SCN9A gene, which causes a significant hyperpolarizing shift in voltage dependence of activation, facilitates channel opening, and increases the amplitude of current produced by Na_v1.7. Small fiber neuropathy (SFN) is a typical pain disorder with burning pain throughout the body, in which electrophysiological analysis of Na_v1.7 channels showed impaired slow inactivation, depolarized fast and slow inactivation, or enhanced resurgent currents [72]. By contrast, Na_v1.7 function mutations in human cause congenital inability to experience pain [77].

7.3 The voltage-gated calcium channel

The VGCCs are a family of membrane proteins which control the influx of calcium ions that trigger neurotransmitter release in response to the depolarization of the presynaptic cell membrane. Calcium ions can not only alter membrane potential but also serve as important signaling entities [78]. VGCCs are expressed on virtually all excitable cells, and their activity is critical for neurotransmitters release, the regulation of neuronal excitability, and intracellular changes including gene induction [79]. VGCCs are classified into high voltage-activated (HVA) or low voltage-activated (LVA) channels based on their voltage dependence of activation [80]. HVA channels are subdivided further based on their pharmacological and biophysical characteristics into L (Ca_v1.1–1.3), N (Ca_v2.2), P/Q (Ca_v2.1), and R-type (Ca_v2.3) [81], and LVA channels are known as T-type channels. HVA channels are complexes of a pore-forming α1 subunit, a transmembrane disulfide-linked complex of α2 and δ subunits, an intracellular β subunit, and in some cases a transmembrane γ subunit [82], while T-type calcium channels are formed by a single α1 subunit [83]. These different subtypes of HVA and LVA channels correspond to ten different α1 subunits, three of which termed Ca_v1, Ca_v2, and Ca_v3 are key determinants of calcium channel subtype [84]. These channels are established and clinically validated drug targets for pain, and their roles and contributions to pain transmission have been extensively reviewed [85].

7.3.1 T-type calcium channels

T-type calcium channel family includes three subtypes, namely, Ca_v3.1, Ca_v3.2, and Ca_v3.3. T-currents have a unique function in neuronal excitability. In comparison with HVA channels, T-type calcium channels can activate at much more negative membrane potentials, inactivate rapidly, deactivate slowly, have small single-channel conductance, and are insensitive to calcium ion antagonist drugs [82]. The large T-type currents are essential for light touch perception, long-term potentiation of synaptic transmission between nociceptive primary afferents, and superficial laminae SP-sensitive neurons of the dorsal horn [86, 87]. Reverse transcription (RT)–PCR and in situ hybridization analyses have shown that the most abundant T-type channels, Ca_v3.2, are expressed in small- and medium-diameter primary afferent neurons as well as neurons from the superficial laminae of the dorsal horn [88]. These Ca_v3.2 T-type channels in primary nociceptors are important regulators of afferent fiber excitability and contribute to peripheral sensitization [89].

7.3.2 Ca_v3.2 T-type calcium channels

The Ca_v3.2 subtype is a particularly attractive analgesic target. An increase in Ca_V3.2 T-type currents is associated with decreased nociceptive threshold, whereas inhibition of Ca_v3.2 channel activity mediates pain relief [90, 91]. A study indicated that intrathecal injection of Ca_v3.2 antisense oligonucleotide but not Ca_v3.1 or Ca_v3.3 antisense oligonucleotide resulted in about an 80% decrease in T-type calcium currents in DRG neurons, and only Ca_v3.2 antisense treatment attenuated nocifensive responses in both naïve and neuropathic pain rats [92]. Several studies validated the potential utility of blocking Ca_v3.2 T-type calcium channels to reduce nociception. For example, in a rat model of paclitaxel-induced peripheral neuropathy, T-type current amplitudes and density in DRG neurons were increased at day 7 after paclitaxel treatment and this was prevented by pretreatment of the specific Ca_v3.2 T-type calcium channel inhibitor ML218 hydrochloride [93]. Selective inhibition of Ca_v3.2 channels reversed hyperexcitability of peripheral nociceptors and alleviated thermal and mechanical hypersensitivity in rodent model of postsurgical pain [94]. However, Ca_v3.2 knock-out mice showed reduced sensitivity to noxious pain but not chronic neuropathic pain [95], which contrasts with the potent analgesic actions of intrathecally delivered Ca_v3.2 channel blockers in neuropathic pain models, suggesting that there is compensation from other types of calcium channels in the afferent fibers of $Ca_v3.2$ null mice that maintain pain transmission [96].

7.3.3 Other calcium channels

Primary afferent neurons express multiple types of VGCCs, P-, N-, L-, R-, T-type, and ancillary α2δ calcium channels have been most extensively studied with regard to chronic pain. N-type calcium channels are enriched at presynaptic nerve terminals where they trigger the release of neurotransmitters [97, 98], and inhibiting N-type channel activity results in reduced neurotransmission and thus analgesia [99, 100]. Moreover, $Ca_v2.2$ channel knock-out mice decreased pain responses in neuropathic and inflammatory pain [101–104]. Besides N-type channels, blockade of L-type and P/Q-type can also prevent and/or attenuate subjective pain as well as primary and/or secondary hyperalgesia and allodynia in a variety of experimental and clinical conditions [105].

The Ca_v α2δ subunit is an important accessory subunit for all HVA calcium channels, and numerous studies point to an important role of α2δ in neuropathic pain. The α2δ-1 mRNA and protein levels are dramatically up-regulated in DRG in several models of neuropathic pain [79], and this increase in α2δ-1 correlates with the onset of allodynia [106, 107]. In clinical practice, the Ca_vα2δ subunit is the key pharmacological target for gabapentinoids (highly effective in the treatment of neuropathic pain) such as gabapentin and pregabalin [108, 109].

8. Neurotransmitters and receptors

8.1 G-protein coupled receptors

G-protein coupled receptor (GPCR) plays an important role in peripheral sensitization. The heterotrimeric GPCRs are the largest, most diverse receptor families in the mammalian cells. GPCRs are integral membrane signaling proteins characterized by a seven-transmembrane-segment architecture. Upon activation of GPCRs, GPCRs associate with distinct classes of heterotrimeric G proteins, composed of α-, β-, and γ-subunits, and molecular cloning has now defined 34 genes encoding G-proteins in humans, 17 encoding α-, 5 encoding β-, and 12 encoding γ-subunits [110, 111]. According to the a-subunits, G proteins are classified into four major classes, namely, Gs, Gi/o, $Gq/_{11}$, and $G_{12/13}$. Stimulation of the Gs subfamily activates adenylyl cyclase whereas stimulation of the Gi subfamily leads to its inhibition. Stimulation of the Gq subfamily activates phospholipase C (PLC), and the G_{12} family is implicated in the regulation of small GTP binding proteins [110].

Through Gα and Gβγ, GPCRs are able to communicate with ligand- and voltage-dependent ion channels in pain pathways [112], including the TRP channels, acid-sensing ion channels (ASICS), and ATP-gated P2X channels, as well as voltage-gated sodium, calcium, and potassium channels [113]. The voltage-gated ion channels are finely tuned by GPCR in excitable cells, and these channels are key molecular transducers of electrical activities, allowing calcium signaling into the cells in response to action potentials or subthreshold depolarizations [114].

In chronic pain conditions, inflammatory mediators released by peripheral tissues and immune cells in response to injury act at GPCRs to sensitize peripheral nociceptors and therefore augment their responses to both noxious and innocuous stimuli. GPCRs can block pain upon targeting opioid, cannabinoid, α2-adrenergic, muscarinic acetylcholine, GABA, Group II and III mGlu, and somatostatin receptors.

8.2 Glutamate

Glutamate is an important excitatory neurotransmitter in the nervous system. There are two classes of the receptors: ionotropic glutamate receptors (iGluRs) and mGluRs. iGluR is a ligand-gated ion channel, whose subtypes are named for the agonist that activates the receptors, including the NMDA, α-amino-3-hydroxy-5-methyl-4-isoxazole propionic acid (AMPA), and kainate receptors (KA) [115]. mGluRs contain eight subtypes of receptors and are divided into three groups: Group I mGluRs (mGluR1 and mGluR5) are coupled to phospholipase C, activate PKC, and release Ca^{2+} from intracellular stores; Group II mGluRs (mGluR2 and mGluR3) and group III mGluRs (mGluR4, mGluR6-8) inhibit adenylyl cyclase activity [116, 117]. Both group II and group III mGluRs are mainly localized on presynaptic terminals.

All subtypes of iGluRs are found on DRG cells and can be transported into central and peripheral terminals by afferent axons. Besides, mGluRs have been identified on peripheral primary afferent fibers and are involved in the processing of peripheral nociception [118]. The excitation of the primary afferent neuron increases glutamate release in the peripheral and central ends of primary afferent neurons [119].

8.2.1 Glutamate and pain

Peripherally applied NMDA and non-NMDA receptor antagonists attenuate or block nociceptive behaviors in several animal models of inflammation pain [120–122]. The fact that injection of NMDA into the masseter muscle potently excites muscle afferent fibers and that local application of NMDA receptor antagonists abolishes glutamate-evoked increase in afferent discharge suggests that activation of peripheral NMDA receptors plays an important role in excitation of muscle afferent fibers [123]. A study showed that injection of glutamate into human masseter and temporalis muscles evoked pain and it could be decreased by co-injection of NMDA antagonist ketamine [124].

Glutamate not only plays an important role in nociception transmission, but also is involved in the inflammation pain and neuropathic pain. Glutamate levels and the number of glutamate receptors elevate during cutaneous or deep tissue inflammation. Peripheral inflammation increases the proportions of both unmyelinated and myelinated nerves expressing iGluRs [125]. Local injection of either NMDA or non-NMDA receptor antagonist significantly reduces thermal hyperalgesia induced by injection of carrageenan into the hind paw or injection of the kaolin/carrageenan into the knee joint, but without affecting joint edema [120]. Activation of group II mGluRs by mGluR2/3 agonists induces analgesia in inflammatory and neuropathic pain models [126, 127]. Activation of Group II mGluRs suppresses prostaglandin E2-induced sensitization of TRPV1 calcium responses in mice [128]. CFA-induced nociceptive behaviors were significantly alleviated by administration of L-AP4, group III mGluR agonist, suggesting that group III mGluRs negatively regulate nociceptive behaviors and pain transmission by lessening neuronal firing rates at the peripheral nerve in inflammation [117]. Group I mGluR antagonists and group II/III mGluR agonists attenuated the enhanced nociception and noxious stimulus-induced glutamate release in the spinal cord dorsal horn in rats of CCI model and injection of CFA into hind paw, suggesting a possible mechanism for their anti-hyperalgesic effects [129].

8.2.2 Ionotropic glutamate receptors

Neurochemical studies indicate that neurotransmitters diffuse across the synaptic cleft (synaptic transmission) as well as diffuse through the extracellular space and affect nearby neurons (non-synaptic communication) in the central nervous system. This is confirmed in a study that the site of action for glutamate can be at the autologous or nearby nerve terminals, and activation of these receptors can lower the activation threshold and increase the excitability of primary afferents [130]. In our experiments [18], we set up repeated antidromic stimulation of T9 nerve branch and recorded the activities from T10 cutaneous nerve branch. Forty minutes after the first antidromic stimulation of the T9 nerve branch, either NMDA receptor antagonist dizocilpine maleate (MK-801) or non-NMDA receptor antagonist 6,7-dinitroquinoxaline-2,3-dione (DNQX) is injected subcutaneously to the receptive field of T10 cutaneous branch, and the enhanced spontaneous discharges in the T10 cutaneous branch caused by stimulation of the T9 nerve branch were significantly blocked. The results indicate that peripheral iGluRs are involved in the activation of peripheral nerves following the antidromic stimulation, and the released glutamate diffuses to the adjacent sensory nerves and activates the adjacent afferents by binding to glutamate receptors located on the nerve terminals. No significant difference was found in effects on the nerve activities between the NMDA and non-NMDA iGluR antagonists, and injection of saline did not produce any effect on the increased discharges of the recorded nerve branch. These results provide us evidence that glutamate may contribute to interactions between peripheral nerve terminals via non-synaptic communication [131]. Cao et al. [132] summarized the evidence that glutamate released from the non-synaptic communication contributes to the nociception in peripheral: (1) electrical stimulation of peripheral nerve can result in the release of glutamate into peripheral tissues; (2) NMDA, AMPA, and KA receptors localize on a large population of myelinated and unmyelinated sensory axons in the peripheral nerves; (3) primary afferents can be excited by the exogenous glutamate and endogenous glutamate; and (4) no synaptic contacts have been reported between two peripheral nerves using morphological approaches.

8.2.3 Glutamate interacts with other receptors

Glutamate receptors may interact with other neurotransmitter receptors in the peripheral to regulate nociception. A study found that peripheral glutamate receptors and TRPV1 receptors may interact to modulate the peripheral sensitization in some deep craniofacial nociceptive afferents [133]. CaMKII, which is persistently activated after NMDA receptor stimulation and phosphorylation of TRPV1, is likely to mediate the interactions between peripheral NMDA and TRPV1 receptors [134]. Glutamate, SP, and CGRP together contribute to the heat hyperalgesia combined with inflammation in the TRPV1-Cre mice [135]. There was a novel concept that tramadol acts as an agonist of TRPV1 [136] and local administration of tramadol blocked the paw licking (nociceptive behavior) in mice induced by glutamate [137].

A few studies on interactions between glutamate and opioid in the periphery have been conducted. A behavioral study has demonstrated that local cutaneous injection of DAMGO, a μ-opioid ligand, ameliorates the nociceptive behaviors caused by local injection of glutamate [138]. Our previous study demonstrated that local application of morphine suppressed the glutamate-evoked excitatory responses of Aδ and C fibers in the rat hairy skin, and this effect was reversed by pretreatment with the opioid receptor antagonist naloxone, suggesting that the effect of morphine on glutamate-evoked activities is mediated through activation of opioid receptors on the peripheral terminals of sensory neurons [139]. Glutamate is released from small diameter afferent fibers by heat stimulation in the periphery or local application of capsaicin, and the glutamate release is regulated by activation of opioid receptors on the peripheral endings of small-diameter afferent fibers [140].

Injection of SP significantly increases the afferent discharge of peripheral sensory nerve endings [25]. A radioimmunoassay study showed that SP contents in the skin and tissues increased after electroacupuncture [141], indicating that SP plays a direct role in the stimulation of skin sensory nerve endings. Our previous study provided electrophysiological evidence for an interaction between SP receptor and glutamate receptor on the fine fiber activities in rat hairy skin, which may be involved in the mechanisms of hyperalgesia. Sub-threshold doses of SP (1 μmol/L, 10 μL) injected subcutaneously into the dorsal hairy skin had no effect on the afferent discharges of either Aδ or C units, while local injection of the submaximal doses of glutamate (10 μmol/L, 10 μL) into the receptive fields increased the afferent discharges of 35% (11/31) of Aδ fibers and 33% (6/18) of C fibers. In addition, glutamate-induced excitatory response was significantly enhanced by coinjection of subthreshold doses of SP [142]. Effects of glutamate and SP on spinal dorsal horn neurons may result from co-release of these two mediators from the same dorsal root afferent terminals [143].

8.3 Opioid

8.3.1 Opioid receptors

Peripheral nerve endings also express a variety of inhibitory neurotransmitter receptors such as opioid, GABA, and cannabinoid receptors. These receptors are related to peripheral sensitization and they may be targets for analgesia drug development. Opioid is known as the most powerful drug for severe pain, including three classic opioid receptors in the central nervous system: μ-(MOR), δ-(DOR), and κ-(KOR) receptors [144]. The existence of the three receptors was confirmed by the identification and sequence analysis of complementary DNA and the selective deletion of opioid receptor genes [145]. In peripheral, opioid receptors are present on the peripheral terminals of thinly myelinated and unmyelinated cutaneous sensory fibers [138]. Opioid agonists can attenuate the excitability of primary afferent neurons and the release of proinflammatory neuropeptides from central and peripheral terminals. Particularly within injured tissue, these events lead to antinociceptive and anti-inflammatory effects [146].

All opioid receptors are members of the rhodopsin class of GPCR, principally, although not exclusively, mediating their effects via the Gi/o pertussis toxin (PTX)-sensitive heterotrimeric G-protein family. After the ligand binds at the receptor, conformational changes allow intracellular coupling of mainly Gi/o proteins to the C-terminus of opioid receptors [147]. The μ-opioid agonists are still the gold standard for the treatment of moderate and severe pain. Agonists of μ-receptors exclusively coupled to inhibitory Gi/o proteins, which is important in anesthesia as they mediate the analgesic and sedative/hypnotic actions [148].

8.3.2 Opioids and pain

Both experimental and clinical studies suggest that peripheral analgesic effects of opioids are predominant under inflammatory conditions, leading to upregulation of opioid receptors on peripheral sensory neurons and to local production of endogenous opioid peptides in immune cells [149–151]. The reason why opioids are predominantly functional under inflammatory conditions is that the opioid-producing cells are recruited in the inflamed tissue but not non-inflamed tissue [152]. In models of peripheral inflammation, local injection of low, systemically inactive doses of μ, δ, and κ-receptor agonists produced analgesia which was dose-dependent, stereospecific, and reversible by selective opioid antagonists [153]. In CFA-induced paw inflammation, MOR mRNA displayed a biphasic upregulation (at 2 h and 96 h), whereas mRNA for DOR remained unchanged, and KOR mRNA showed a peak at 12 h [154, 155]. In addition, human studies indicated that local application of opioid agonists are beneficial in patients with visceral and neuropathic pain as these drugs have analgesic efficacy and less side-effects because they do not readily cross the blood-brain barrier [48, 156].

8.3.3 Opioid-induced hyperalgesia

Unexpectedly, a large number of studies have demonstrated that opioids can elicit hyperalgesia and allodynia [157]. Opioid-induced hyperalgesia (OIH) may be associated with analgesic tolerance. OIH refers usually to the development of hypersensitivity to painful stimuli observed upon chronic opioid administration. Different mechanisms have been identified for this process including sensitization of primary afferent neurons and enhanced release of glutamate by these primary afferents, hyperexcitability of second order neurons to excitatory neurotransmitters, and up-regulation of nociceptive neuromodulators by descending pain controls [158, 159]. A lot of evidence suggests that MOR antagonists might reduce opioid analgesia [160]. However, the co-administration of methylnaltrexone bromide, a peripherally restricted MOR antagonist, was sufficient to abolish morphine tolerance and OIH without diminishing antinociception in perioperative and chronic pain models [161].

8.3.4 Other inhibitory receptors

Endogenous inhibitory receptors play a crucial part in the management of pain. Peripheral sensory neurons exhibit a large number of receptors that mediate inhibition of neuronal activity, and the agonists of these receptors produce antinociception. Application of either $GABA_A$ or $GABA_B$ receptor agonists attenuated the colonic afferent response to colon stretch. Conversely, $GABA_A$ and $GABA_B$ receptor antagonists increased the stretch response. These results suggest that GABA receptors are present and functional in the peripheral terminals of colonic afferents, and activation of these receptors via endogenous GABA release contributes to the suppression of colonic afferent excitability and visceral nociception without the central nervous system [162]. The antinociceptive effects of cannabinoids were confirmed in preclinical models of inflammatory, cancer, and neuropathic pain and in several human studies [163]. In an animal electrophysiological model similar to our previous studies [164], somatostatin inhibited the cross excitation between nerve terminals involved in peripheral hyperalgesia and had a peripheral analgesic effect [164]. The somatostatin and its receptors exerted a tonic inhibitory control over peripheral nociceptors, especially the peripheral nerve terminals of small-diameter cutaneous afferent fibers [165].

9. Conclusion

Based on the up-to-date studies in peripheral sensitization, we establish the essential roles of inflammation mediators, neurotransmitters, and their receptors in this process, expecting to provide a new prospect of analgesics on peripheral targets in pain management. Noxious stimuli can excite the peripheral endings of primary sensory afferents, through activation of voltage-gated ion channels and/or ligand-gated receptors that increase the number of action potentials, leading to peripheral sensitization. Many inflammation mediators and neurotransmitters participate in the peripheral sensitization. Therefore, these chemicals provide enormous options for pain intervention of peripheral origin. Topically administered drugs such as lidocaine and capsaicin in patches, capsaicin in cream, and creams containing anti-depressants (i.e., doxepin and amitriptyline) act locally in tissues through specific receptors and/or ion channels [166]. Topical drug delivery focuses on peripheral mechanisms and not only reaches greater concentrations in the region where it is applied, but also produces fewer side-effects along with greatly enhanced efficacy. Considering the unspecific and multifaceted function of chemicals involved in the peripheral sensitization, it is crucial to select the most suitable and specific targets to treat certain pain disease in clinic.

Beyond the peripheral sensitization, changes in the central nervous system neurons also play an essential role in the nociception process. Multiple lines of evidence show that central sensitization, produced following intense peripheral noxious stimuli, tissue injury, or nerve damage, is involved in diverse pain conditions, such as myofascial pain syndromes, idiopathic low back pain, and chronic pelvic pain [167]. Given the complexity and diversity of peripheral and central mechanisms of various pain conditions, it needs further investigation to figure out the specific mechanisms of pain symptoms and identify the most effective pain therapies in future.

Acknowledgements

This work was supported by the National Natural Science Foundation of China (81971049, 81671097).

Author details

Si-Qi Wei, Zhuo-Ying Tao, Yang Xue and Dong-Yuan Cao*
Key Laboratory of Shaanxi Province for Craniofacial Precision Medicine Research, Research Center of Stomatology, Xi'an Jiaotong University College of Stomatology, Xi'an, Shaanxi, P.R. China

*Address all correspondence to: dongyuan_cao@hotmail.com

References

[1] Campbell JN, Meyer RA. Mechanisms of neuropathic pain. Neuron. 2006;**52**(1):77-92

[2] Berta T, Qadri Y, Tan PH, Ji RR. Targeting dorsal root ganglia and primary sensory neurons for the treatment of chronic pain. Expert Opinion on Therapeutic Targets. 2017;**21**(7):695-703

[3] Basbaum AI, Bautista DM, Scherrer G, Julius D. Cellular and molecular mechanisms of pain. Cell. 2009;**139**(2):267-284

[4] Woolf CJ. Evidence for a central component of post-injury pain hypersensitivity. Nature. 1983;**306**(5944):686-688

[5] Ashmawi HA, Freire GMG. Peripheral and central sensitization. Revista Dor. 2016;**17**(Suppl 1):S31-S34

[6] Dunteman ED. Targeted peripheral analgesics in chronic pain syndromes. Practical Pain Management. 2005;**5**(5)

[7] Gold MS, Gebhart GF. Nociceptor sensitization in pain pathogenesis. Nature Medicine. 2010;**16**(11):1248-1257

[8] Raja SN, Meyer RA, Campbell JN. Peripheral mechanisms of somatic pain. Anesthesiology. 1988;**68**(4):571-590

[9] Tracey WD Jr. Nociception. Current Biology. 2017;**27**(4):R129-R133

[10] Vardeh D, Naranjo JF. Peripheral and central sensitization. Pain Medicine. 2017:15-17

[11] Gangadharan V, Kuner R. Pain hypersensitivity mechanisms at a glance. Disease Models & Mechanisms. 2013;**6**(4):889-895

[12] Schaible HG, Ebersberger A, Natura G. Update on peripheral mechanisms of pain: Beyond prostaglandins and cytokines. Arthritis Research & Therapy. 2011;**13**(2):210

[13] Yekkirala AS, Roberson DP, Bean BP, Woolf CJ. Breaking barriers to novel analgesic drug development. Nature Reviews. Drug Discovery. 2017;**16**(8):545-564

[14] Zollner C, Mousa SA, Fischer O, Rittner HL, Shaqura M, Brack A, et al. Chronic morphine use does not induce peripheral tolerance in a rat model of inflammatory pain. The Journal of Clinical Investigation. 2008;**118**(3):1065-1073

[15] Weyer-Menkhoff I, Lotsch J. Human pharmacological approaches to TRP-ion-channel-based analgesic drug development. Drug Discovery Today. 2018;**23**(12):2003-2012

[16] Gregory NS, Harris AL, Robinson CR, Dougherty PM, Fuchs PN, Sluka KA. An overview of animal models of pain: Disease models and outcome measures. The Journal of Pain. 2013;**14**(11):1255-1269

[17] Zhao Y, Shi WC, Wang HS, Jia FY, Huang QE. Information transmission between two sensory nerve endings in rats. Journal of Xi'an Medical University. 1996;**17**(02):140-142

[18] Cao DY, You HJ, Zhao Y, Guo Y, Wang HS, Nielsen LA, et al. Involvement of peripheral ionotropic glutamate receptors in activation of cutaneous branches of spinal dorsal rami following antidromic electrical stimulation of adjacent afferent nerves in rats. Brain Research Bulletin. 2007;**72**(1):10-17

[19] Lynn B, Carpenter SE. Primary afferent units from the hairy skin of the rat hind limb. Brain Research. 1982;**238**(1):29-43

[20] Sun QX, Zhang Y, Zhao Y, Zhang SH, Shi WC, Wang HS. Changes of mechano-receptive properties of Adelta-fibers of adjacent spinal segments after antidromical electrical stimulation of dorsal cutaneous nerve. Acupunct Research. 2003;**28**(02):102-110

[21] Zhang SH, Zhao Y, Sun QX, Shi WC, Wang HS. The effect of electrical stimulation of the cutaneous nerve of the adjacent spinal segment on afferent discharges of C-mechanoreceptive units in rats. Acupuncture Research. 2001;**26**(1):5-9

[22] Zhang SH, Sun QX, Seltzer Z, Cao DY, Wang HS, Chen Z, et al. Paracrine-like excitation of low-threshold mechanoceptive C-fibers innervating rat hairy skin is mediated by substance P via NK-1 receptors. Brain Research Bulletin. 2008;**75**(1):138-145

[23] Sun QX, Zhao Y, Zhang SH, Shi WC, Wang HS. Discharge changes of Aβ-fibers of the dorsal cutaneous branch in spinal nerve evoked by electrical stimulation of adjacent spinal segments. Journal of the Fourth Military Medical University. 2002;**23**(1):23

[24] Li JH, He PY, Fan DN, Alemujiang D, Huo FQ, Zhao Y, et al. Peripheral ionotropic glutamate receptors contribute to Fos expression increase in the spinal cord through antidromic electrical stimulation of sensory nerves. Neuroscience Letters. 2018;**678**:1-7

[25] Shi WC, Zhao Y, Zhang BZ. The role of substance P and histamine in the information transmmation along channels. Chinese Acupuncture & Moxibustion. 1995;**04**:33-35

[26] Jia J, Zhao Y, Shi WC, Wang HS, Guo Y. Effect of electrical stimulation of the dorsal cutaneous branches of spinal nerve on the discharge activity of remote mechanoreceptive units in rats. Acta Physiologica. 2002;**02**:125-128

[27] Zhao Y, Shi WC, Wang HS, Jia FY. Neurokiinin A and information transmission along channels. Journal of Xi'an Jiaotong University. 1997;**02**:149-151

[28] Bhave G, RWt G. Posttranslational mechanisms of peripheral sensitization. Journal of Neurobiology. 2004;**61**(1):88-106

[29] Devesa I, Ferrandiz-Huertas C, Mathivanan S, Wolf C, Lujan R, Changeux JP, et al. alphaCGRP is essential for algesic exocytotic mobilization of TRPV1 channels in peptidergic nociceptors. Proceedings of the National Academy of Sciences of the United States of America. 2014;**111**(51):18345-18350

[30] Ma W, Eisenach JC. Morphological and pharmacological evidence for the role of peripheral prostaglandins in the pathogenesis of neuropathic pain. The European Journal of Neuroscience. 2002;**15**(6):1037-1047

[31] Hucho T, Levine JD. Signaling pathways in sensitization: Toward a nociceptor cell biology. Neuron. 2007;**55**(3):365-376

[32] Syriatowicz JP, Hu D, Walker JS, Tracey DJ. Hyperalgesia due to nerve injury: Role of prostaglandins. Neuroscience. 1999;**94**(2):587-594

[33] Kroin JS, Buvanendran A, Watts DE, Saha C, Tuman KJ. Upregulation of cerebrospinal fluid and peripheral prostaglandin E2 in a rat postoperative pain model. Anesthesia and Analgesia. 2006;**103**(2):334-343. Table of contents

[34] Villarreal CF, Funez MI, Cunha Fde Q, Parada CA, Ferreira SH. The long-lasting sensitization of primary afferent nociceptors induced by inflammation involves prostanoid and dopaminergic systems in mice. Pharmacology, Biochemistry, and Behavior. 2013;**103**(3):678-683

[35] Hall JM. Bradykinin receptors. General Pharmacology. 1997;**28**(1):1-6

[36] Regoli D, Nsa Allogho S, Rizzi A, Gobeil FJ. Bradykinin receptors and their antagonists. European Journal of Pharmacology. 1998;**348**(1):1-10

[37] Schuelert N, Just S, Corradini L, Kuelzer R, Bernloehr C, Doods H. The bradykinin B1 receptor antagonist BI113823 reverses inflammatory hyperalgesia by desensitization of peripheral and spinal neurons. European Journal of Pain. 2015;**19**(1):132-142

[38] Burgess GM, Mullaney I, McNeill M, Dunn PM, Rang HP. Second messengers involved in the mechanism of action of bradykinin in sensory neurons in culture. The Journal of Neuroscience. 1989;**9**(9):3314-3325

[39] Levy D, Zochodne DW. Increased mRNA expression of the B1 and B2 bradykinin receptors and antinociceptive effects of their antagonists in an animal model of neuropathic pain. Pain. 2000;**86**(3):265-271

[40] Mayer S, Izydorczyk I, Reeh PW, Grubb BD. Bradykinin-induced nociceptor sensitisation to heat depends on cox-1 and cox-2 in isolated rat skin. Pain. 2007;**130**(1-2):14-24

[41] Samanta A, Hughes TET, Moiseenkova-Bell VY. Transient receptor potential (TRP) channels. Sub-Cellular Biochemistry. 2018;**87**:141-165

[42] Liao M, Cao E, Julius D, Cheng Y. Structure of the TRPV1 ion channel determined by electron cryo-microscopy. Nature. 2013;**504**(7478):107-112

[43] Tominaga M, Caterina MJ, Malmberg AB, Rosen TA, Gilbert H, Skinner K, et al. The cloned capsaicin receptor integrates multiple pain-producing stimuli. Neuron. 1998;**21**(3):531-543

[44] Caterina MJ, Schumacher MA, Tominaga M, Rosen TA, Levine JD, Julius D. The capsaicin receptor: A heat-activated ion channel in the pain pathway. Nature. 1997;**389**(6653):816-824

[45] Simone DA, Baumann TK, LaMotte RH. Dose-dependent pain and mechanical hyperalgesia in humans after intradermal injection of capsaicin. Pain. 1989;**38**(1):99-107

[46] LaMotte RH, Shain CN, Simone DA, Tsai EF. Neurogenic hyperalgesia: Psychophysical studies of underlying mechanisms. Journal of Neurophysiology. 1991;**66**(1):190-211

[47] Okun A, DeFelice M, Eyde N, Ren J, Mercado R, King T, et al. Transient inflammation-induced ongoing pain is driven by TRPV1 sensitive afferents. Molecular Pain. 2011;7:4

[48] Suh YG, Oh U. Activation and activators of TRPV1 and their pharmaceutical implication. Current Pharmaceutical Design. 2005;**11**(21):2687-2698

[49] Warwick CA, Shutov LP, Shepherd AJ, Mohapatra DP, Usachev YM. Mechanisms underlying mechanical sensitization induced by complement C5a: The roles of macrophages, TRPV1, and calcitonin gene-related peptide receptors. Pain. 2019;**160**(3):702-711

[50] Wang C, Gu L, Ruan Y, Gegen T, Yu L, Zhu C, et al. Pirt together with TRPV1 is involved in the regulation of neuropathic pain. Neural Plasticity. 2018;**2018**:4861491

[51] Matheny SA, Chen C, Kortum RL, Razidlo GL, Lewis RE, White MA. Ras regulates assembly of mitogenic signalling complexes through

the effector protein IMP. Nature. 2004;**427**(6971):256-260

[52] Sisignano M, Bennett DL, Geisslinger G, Scholich K. TRP-channels as key integrators of lipid pathways in nociceptive neurons. Progress in Lipid Research. 2014;**53**:93-107

[53] Song C, Liu P, Zhao Q, Guo S, Wang G. TRPV1 channel contributes to remifentanil-induced postoperative hyperalgesia via regulation of NMDA receptor trafficking in dorsal root ganglion. Journal of Pain Research. 2019;**12**:667-677

[54] Mathivanan S, Devesa I, Changeux JP, Ferrer-Montiel A. Bradykinin induces TRPV1 exocytotic recruitment in peptidergic nociceptors. Frontiers in Pharmacology. 2016;**7**:178

[55] Wang Y, Feng C, He H, He J, Wang J, Li X, et al. Sensitization of TRPV1 receptors by TNF-alpha orchestrates the development of vincristine-induced pain. Oncology Letters. 2018;**15**(4):5013-5019

[56] Rukwied R, Schley M, Forsch E, Obreja O, Dusch M, Schmelz M. Nerve growth factor-evoked nociceptor sensitization in pig skin in vivo. Journal of Neuroscience Research. 2010;**88**(9):2066-2072

[57] Saloman JL, Chung MK, Ro JY. P2X(3) and TRPV1 functionally interact and mediate sensitization of trigeminal sensory neurons. Neuroscience. 2013;**232**:226-238

[58] Chung MK, Lee J, Joseph J, Saloman J, Ro JY. Peripheral group I metabotropic glutamate receptor activation leads to muscle mechanical hyperalgesia through TRPV1 phosphorylation in the rat. The Journal of Pain. 2015;**16**(1):67-76

[59] Wang Y, Gao Y, Tian Q, Deng Q, Wang Y, Zhou T, et al. TRPV1 SUMOylation regulates nociceptive signaling in models of inflammatory pain. Nature Communications. 2018;**9**(1):1529

[60] Bandell M, Story GM, Hwang SW, Viswanath V, Eid SR, Petrus MJ, et al. Noxious cold ion channel TRPA1 is activated by pungent compounds and bradykinin. Neuron. 2004;**41**(6):849-857

[61] Moparthi L, Survery S, Kreir M, Simonsen C, Kjellbom P, Högestätt ED, et al. Human TRPA1 is intrinsically cold- and chemosensitive with and without its N-terminal ankyrin repeat domain. Proceedings of the National Academy of Sciences of the United States of America. 2014;**111**(47):16901-16906

[62] Brackley AD, Gomez R, Guerrero KA, Akopian AN, Glucksman MJ, Du J, et al. A-kinase anchoring protein 79/150 scaffolds transient receptor potential A 1 phosphorylation and sensitization by metabotropic glutamate receptor activation. Scientific Reports. 2017;7(1):1842

[63] Zakharian E, Cao C, Rohacs T. Gating of transient receptor potential melastatin 8 (TRPM8) channels activated by cold and chemical agonists in planar lipid bilayers. The Journal of Neuroscience. 2010;**30**(37):12526-12534

[64] Moqrich A, Hwang SW, Earley TJ, Petrus MJ, Murray AN, Spencer KS, et al. Impaired thermosensation in mice lacking TRPV3, a heat and camphor sensor in the skin. Science. 2005;**307**(5714):1468-1472

[65] Alessandri-Haber N, Yeh JJ, Boyd AE, Parada CA, Chen X, Reichling DB, et al. Hypotonicity induces TRPV4-mediated nociception in rat. Neuron. 2003;**39**(3):497-511

[66] Levine JD, Alessandri-Haber N. TRP channels: Targets for the relief of

pain. Biochimica et Biophysica Acta. 2007;**1772**(8):989-1003

[67] Toledo-Aral JJ, Moss BL, He ZJ, Koszowski AG, Whisenand T, Levinson SR, et al. Identification of PN1, a predominant voltage-dependent sodium channel expressed principally in peripheral neurons. Proceedings of the National Academy of Sciences of the United States of America. 1997;**94**(4):1527-1532

[68] Kopsky DJ, Keppel Hesselink JM. Topical phenytoin for the treatment of neuropathic pain. Journal of Pain Research. 2017;**10**:469-473

[69] Weiss J, Pyrski M, Jacobi E, Bufe B, Willnecker V, Schick B, et al. Loss-of-function mutations in sodium channel Nav1.7 cause anosmia. Nature. 2011;**472**(7342):186-190

[70] Black J, Frézel N, Dib-Hajj S, Waxman S. Expression of Nav1.7 in DRG neurons extends from peripheral terminals in the skin to central preterminal branches and terminals in the dorsal horn. Molecular Pain. 2012;**8**:82

[71] Chang W, Berta T, Kim YH, Lee S, Lee SY, Ji RR. Expression and role of voltage-gated sodium channels in human dorsal root ganglion neurons with special focus on Nav1.7, species differences, and regulation by paclitaxel. Neuroscience Bulletin. 2018;**34**(1):4-12

[72] Habib AM, Wood JN, Cox JJ. Sodium channels and pain. Handbook of Experimental Pharmacology. 2015;**227**:39-56

[73] Nassar MA, Stirling LC, Forlani G, Baker MD, Matthews EA, Dickenson AH, et al. Nociceptor-specific gene deletion reveals a major role for Nav1.7 (PN1) in acute and inflammatory pain. Proceedings of the National Academy of Sciences of the United States of America. 2004;**101**(34):12706-12711

[74] Minett MS, Falk S, Santana-Varela S, Bogdanov YD, Nassar MA, Heegaard AM, et al. Pain without nociceptors? Nav1.7-independent pain mechanisms. Cell Reports. 2014;**6**(2):301-312

[75] Black JA, Liu S, Tanaka M, Cummins TR, Waxman SG. Changes in the expression of tetrodotoxin-sensitive sodium channels within dorsal root ganglia neurons in inflammatory pain. Pain. 2004;**108**(3):237-247

[76] Minett MS, Pereira V, Sikandar S, Matsuyama A, Lolignier S, Kanellopoulos AH, et al. Endogenous opioids contribute to insensitivity to pain in humans and mice lacking sodium channel Nav1.7. Nature Communications. 2015;**6**(1)

[77] Ahmad S, Dahllund L, Eriksson AB, Hellgren D, Karlsson U, Lund PE, et al. A stop codon mutation in SCN9A causes lack of pain sensation. Human Molecular Genetics. 2007;**16**(17):2114-2121

[78] Clapham DE. Calcium signaling. Cell. 2007;**131**(6):1047-1058

[79] Yusaf SP, Goodman J, Pinnock RD, Dixon AK, Lee K. Expression of voltage-gated calcium channel subunits in rat dorsal root ganglion neurons. Neuroscience Letters. 2001;**311**(2):137-141

[80] Bean BP. Classes of calcium channels in vertebrate cells. Annual Review of Physiology. 1989;**51**:367-384

[81] Nowycky MC, Fox AP, Tsien RW. Three types of neuronal calcium channel with different calcium agonist sensitivity. Nature. 1985;**316**(6027):440-443

[82] Catterall WA. Structure and regulation of voltage-gated Ca^{2+} channels. Annual Review of Cell

and Developmental Biology. 2000;**16**:521-555

[83] Catterall WA. Voltage-gated calcium channels. Cold Spring Harbor Perspectives in Biology. 2011;**3**(8):a003947

[84] Catterall WA, Perez-Reyes E, Snutch TP, Striessnig J. International Union of Pharmacology. XLVIII. Nomenclature and structure-function relationships of voltage-gated calcium channels. Pharmacological Reviews. 2005;**57**(4):411-425

[85] Bourinet E, Altier C, Hildebrand ME, Trang T, Salter MW, Zamponi GW. Calcium-permeable ion channels in pain signaling. Physiological Reviews. 2014;**94**(1):81-140

[86] Dubreuil AS, Boukhaddaoui H, Desmadryl G, Martinez-Salgado C, Moshourab R, Lewin GR, et al. Role of T-type calcium current in identified D-hair mechanoreceptor neurons studied in vitro. The Journal of Neuroscience. 2004;**24**(39):8480-8484

[87] Ikeda H, Heinke B, Ruscheweyh R, Sandkuhler J. Synaptic plasticity in spinal lamina I projection neurons that mediate hyperalgesia. Science. 2003;**299**(5610):1237-1240

[88] Talley EM, Cribbs LL, Lee JH, Daud A, Perez-Reyes E, Bayliss DA. Differential distribution of three members of a gene family encoding low voltage-activated (T-type) calcium channels. The Journal of Neuroscience. 1999;**19**(6):1895-1911

[89] Nelson MT, Todorovic SM. Is there a role for T-type calcium channels in peripheral and central pain sensitization? Molecular Neurobiology. 2006;**34**(3):243-248

[90] Todorovic SM, Jevtovic-Todorovic V. T-type voltage-gated calcium channels as targets for the development of novel pain therapies. British Journal of Pharmacology. 2011;**163**(3):484-495

[91] Waxman SG, Zamponi GW. Regulating excitability of peripheral afferents: Emerging ion channel targets. Nature Neuroscience. 2014;**17**(2):153-163

[92] Bourinet E, Alloui A, Monteil A, Barrere C, Couette B, Poirot O, et al. Silencing of the Cav3.2 T-type calcium channel gene in sensory neurons demonstrates its major role in nociception. The EMBO Journal. 2005;**24**(2):315-324

[93] Li Y, Tatsui CE, Rhines LD, North RY, Harrison DS, Cassidy RM, et al. Dorsal root ganglion neurons become hyperexcitable and increase expression of voltage-gated T-type calcium channels (Cav3.2) in paclitaxel-induced peripheral neuropathy. Pain. 2017;**158**(3):417-429

[94] Joksimovic SL, Joksimovic SM, Tesic V, Garcia-Caballero A, Feseha S, Zamponi GW, et al. Selective inhibition of CaV3.2 channels reverses hyperexcitability of peripheral nociceptors and alleviates postsurgical pain. Science Signaling. 2018;**11**(545)

[95] Choi S, Na HS, Kim J, Lee J, Lee S, Kim D, et al. Attenuated pain responses in mice lacking Ca(V)3.2 T-type channels. Genes, Brain, and Behavior. 2007;**6**(5):425-431

[96] Simms BA, Zamponi GW. Neuronal voltage-gated calcium channels: Structure, function, and dysfunction. Neuron. 2014;**82**(1):24-45

[97] Westenbroek RE, Hell JW, Warner C, Dubel SJ, Snutch TP, Catterall WA. Biochemical properties and subcellular distribution of an N-type calcium channel alpha 1 subunit. Neuron. 1992;**9**(6):1099-1115

[98] Wheeler DB, Randall A, Tsien RW. Roles of N-type and Q-type Ca^{2+} channels in supporting hippocampal synaptic transmission. Science. 1994;**264**(5155):107-111

[99] Altier C, Dale CS, Kisilevsky AE, Chapman K, Castiglioni AJ, Matthews EA, et al. Differential role of N-type calcium channel splice isoforms in pain. The Journal of Neuroscience. 2007;**27**(24):6363-6373

[100] Pathirathna S, Brimelow BC, Jagodic MM, Krishnan K, Jiang X, Zorumski CF, et al. New evidence that both T-type calcium channels and GABAA channels are responsible for the potent peripheral analgesic effects of 5alpha-reduced neuroactive steroids. Pain. 2005;**114**(3):429-443

[101] Kim C, Jun K, Lee T, Kim SS, McEnery MW, Chin H, et al. Altered nociceptive response in mice deficient in the alpha(1B) subunit of the voltage-dependent calcium channel. Molecular and Cellular Neurosciences. 2001;**18**(2):235-245

[102] Saegusa H, Kurihara T, Zong S, Kazuno A, Matsuda Y, Nonaka T, et al. Suppression of inflammatory and neuropathic pain symptoms in mice lacking the N-type Ca^{2+} channel. The EMBO Journal. 2001;**20**(10):2349-2356

[103] Brittain JM, Duarte DB, Wilson SM, Zhu W, Ballard C, Johnson PL, et al. Suppression of inflammatory and neuropathic pain by uncoupling CRMP-2 from the presynaptic Ca^{2+} channel complex. Nature Medicine. 2011;**17**(7):822-829

[104] Shao PP, Ye F, Chakravarty PK, Varughese DJ, Herrington JB, Dai G, et al. Aminopiperidine sulfonamide Cav2.2 channel inhibitors for the treatment of chronic pain. Journal of Medicinal Chemistry. 2012;**55**(22):9847-9855

[105] Vanegas H, Schaible H. Effects of antagonists to high-threshold calcium channels upon spinal mechanisms of pain, hyperalgesia and allodynia. Pain. 2000;**85**(1-2):9-18

[106] Bauer CS, Nieto-Rostro M, Rahman W, Tran-Van-Minh A, Ferron L, Douglas L, et al. The increased trafficking of the calcium channel subunit alpha2delta-1 to presynaptic terminals in neuropathic pain is inhibited by the alpha2delta ligand pregabalin. The Journal of Neuroscience. 2009;**29**(13):4076-4088

[107] Newton RA, Bingham S, Case PC, Sanger GJ, Lawson SN. Dorsal root ganglion neurons show increased expression of the calcium channel alpha2delta-1 subunit following partial sciatic nerve injury. Brain Research. Molecular Brain Research. 2001;**95**(1-2):1-8

[108] Field MJ, Li Z, Schwarz JB. Ca^{2+} channel alpha2-delta ligands for the treatment of neuropathic pain. Journal of Medicinal Chemistry. 2007;**50**(11):2569-2575

[109] Wiffen PJ, Derry S, Bell RF, Rice AS, Tolle TR, Phillips T, et al. Gabapentin for chronic neuropathic pain in adults. Cochrane Database of Systematic Reviews. 2017;**6**:CD007938

[110] Hur EM, Kim KT. G protein-coupled receptor signalling and cross-talk achieving rapidity and specificity. Cell Signaling. 2002;**14**(5):397-405

[111] Li H, Wang R, Lu Y, Xu X, Ni J. Targeting G protein-coupled receptor for pain management. Brain Circulation. 2017;**3**(2):109-113

[112] Stone LS, Molliver DC. In search of analgesia: Emerging roles of GPCRs in pain. Molecular Interventions. 2009;**9**(5):234-251

[113] Sadeghi M, McArthur JR, Finol-Urdaneta RK, Adams DJ. Analgesic conopeptides targeting G protein-coupled receptors reduce excitability of sensory neurons. Neuropharmacology. 2017;**127**:116-123

[114] Altier C. GPCR and voltage-gated calcium channels (VGCC) signaling complexes. Sub-Cellular Biochemistry. 2012;**63**:241-262

[115] Willis WD. Role of neurotransmitters in sensitization of pain responses. Annals of the New York Academy of Sciences. 2001;**933**:142-156

[116] Conn PJ, Pin JP. Pharmacology and functions of metabotropic glutamate receptors. Annual Review of Pharmacology and Toxicology. 1997;**37**:205-237

[117] Park EH, Lee SW, Moon SW, Suh HR, Kim YI, Han HC. Activation of peripheral group III metabotropic glutamate receptors inhibits pain transmission by decreasing neuronal excitability in the CFA-inflamed knee joint. Neuroscience Letters. 2019;**694**:111-115

[118] Carlton SM. Peripheral excitatory amino acids. Current Opinion in Pharmacology. 2001;**1**(1):52-56

[119] deGroot J, Zhou S, Carlton SM. Peripheral glutamate release in the hindpaw following low and high intensity sciatic stimulation. Neuroreport. 2000;**11**(3):497-502

[120] Omote K, Kawamata T, Kawamata M, Namiki A. Formalin-induced release of excitatory amino acids in the skin of the rat hindpaw. Brain Research. 1998;**787**(1):161-164

[121] Lawand NB, Willis WD, Westlund KN. Excitatory amino acid receptor involvement in peripheral nociceptive transmission in rats. European Journal of Pharmacology. 1997;**324**(2-3):169-177

[122] Carlton SM, Zhou S, Coggeshall RE. Evidence for the interaction of glutamate and NK1 receptors in the periphery. Brain Research. 1998;**790**(1-2):160-169

[123] Dong XD, Mann MK, Sessle BJ, Arendt-Nielsen L, Svensson P, Cairns BE. Sensitivity of rat temporalis muscle afferent fibers to peripheral N-methyl-D-aspartate receptor activation. Neuroscience. 2006;**141**(2):939-945

[124] Castrillon EE, Cairns BE, Wang K, Arendt-Nielsen L, Svensson P. Comparison of glutamate-evoked pain between the temporalis and masseter muscles in men and women. Pain. 2012;**153**(4):823-829

[125] Carlton SM, Zhou S, Coggeshall RE.Peripheral GABA(A) receptors: Evidence for peripheral primary afferent depolarization. Neuroscience. 1999;**93**(2):713-722

[126] Fisher K, Coderre TJ. The contribution of metabotropic glutamate receptors (mGluRs) to formalin-induced nociception. Pain. 1996;**68**(2-3):255-263

[127] Sharpe EF, Kingston AE, Lodge D, Monn JA, Headley PM. Systemic pre-treatment with a group II mGlu agonist, LY379268, reduces hyperalgesia in vivo. British Journal of Pharmacology. 2002;**135**(5):1255-1262

[128] Sheahan TD, Valtcheva MV, McIlvried LA, Pullen MY, Baranger DAA, Gereau RW. Metabotropic glutamate receptor 2/3 (mGluR2/3) activation suppresses TRPV1 sensitization in mouse, but not human. Sensory Neurons. eNeuro. 2018;**5**(2):e0412-e0417

[129] Kumar N, Laferriere A, Yu JS, Poon T, Coderre TJ. Metabotropic glutamate receptors (mGluRs) regulate noxious stimulus-induced glutamate release in the spinal cord dorsal horn of rats with neuropathic and inflammatory pain. Journal of Neurochemistry. 2010;**114**(1):281-290

[130] Miller KE, Hoffman EM, Sutharshan M, Schechter R. Glutamate pharmacology and metabolism in peripheral primary afferents: Physiological and pathophysiological mechanisms. Pharmacology & Therapeutics. 2011;**130**(3):283-309

[131] Cao DY, Guo Y, Zhang Q, Tian YL, Wang HS, Zhao Y. Effects of glutamate on the afferent discharges of dorsal cutaneous sensory nerves in rats. Neuroscience Bulletin. 2005;**21**(2):111-116

[132] Cao DY, Zhao Y, GUO Y, Pickar JG. Glutamate receptors involved in interaction between peripheral nerve terminals. In: TE PBW, editor. Amino Acid Receptor Research. 2008. pp. 309-327

[133] Lam DK, Sessle BJ, Glutamate HJW. Capsaicin effects on trigeminal nociception I: Activation and peripheral sensitization of deep craniofacial nociceptive afferents. Brain Research. 2009;**1251**:48-59

[134] Petrenko AB, Yamakura T, Baba H, Shimoji K. The role of N-methyl-D-aspartate (NMDA) receptors in pain: A review. Anesthesia and Analgesia. 2003;**97**(4):1108-1116

[135] Rogoz K, Andersen HH, Kullander K, Lagerstrom MC. Glutamate, substance P, and calcitonin gene-related peptide cooperate in inflammation-induced heat hyperalgesia. Molecular Pharmacology. 2014;**85**(2):322-334

[136] Marincsak R, Toth BI, Czifra G, Szabo T, Kovacs L, Biro T. The analgesic drug, tramadol, acts as an agonist of the transient receptor potential vanilloid-1. Anesthesia and Analgesia. 2008;**106**(6):1890-1896

[137] Wang JT, Chung CC, Whitehead RA, Schwarz SK, Ries CR, MacLeod BA. Effects of local tramadol administration on peripheral glutamate-induced nociceptive behaviour in mice. Canadian Journal of Anaesthesia. 2010;**57**(7):659-663

[138] Coggeshall RE, Zhou S, Carlton SM. Opioid receptors on peripheral sensory axons. Brain Research. 1997;**764**(1-2):126-132

[139] Tian YL, Guo Y, Cao DY, Zhang Q, Wang HS, Zhao Y. Local application of morphine suppresses glutamate-evoked activities of C and Aδ afferent fibers in rat hairy skin. Brain Research. 2005;**1059**(1):28-34

[140] Jin YH, Nishioka H, Wakabayashi K, Fujita T, Yonehara N. Effect of morphine on the release of excitatory amino acids in the rat hind instep: Pain is modulated by the interaction between the peripheral opioid and glutamate systems. Neuroscience. 2006;**138**(4):1329-1339

[141] Cao DY, Niu HZ, Zhao Y, Du JQ, Zhu ZL. Stimulation of acupoint induce release of substance P and through primary afferent reflex. Chinese Acupuncture & Moxibustion. 2001;**21**(10):623-625

[142] Zhang Q, Zhao Y, Guo Y, Cao DY, Tian YL, Yao FR, et al. Electrophysiological evidence for the interaction of substance P and glutamate on Adelta and C afferent fibre activity in rat hairy skin. Clinical and Experimental Pharmacology & Physiology. 2006;**33**(12):1128-1133

[143] De Biasi S, Rustioni A. Glutamate and substance P coexist in primary afferent terminals in the superficial

laminae of spinal cord. Proceedings of the National Academy of Sciences of the United States of America. 1988;**85**(20):7820-7824

[144] Lord JA, Waterfield AA, Hughes J, Kosterlitz HW. Endogenous opioid peptides: Multiple agonists and receptors. Nature. 1977;**267**(5611):495-499

[145] Law PY, Reggio PH, Loh HH. Opioid receptors: Toward separation of analgesic from undesirable effects. Trends in Biochemical Sciences. 2013;**38**(6):275-282

[146] Stein C, Schafer M, Machelska H. Attacking pain at its source: New perspectives on opioids. Nature Medicine. 2003;**9**(8):1003-1008

[147] Herlitze S, Garcia DE, Mackie K, Hille B, Scheuer T, Catterall WA. Modulation of Ca^{2+} channels by G-protein beta gamma subunits. Nature. 1996;**380**(6571):258-262

[148] Connor M, Christie MD. Opioid receptor signalling mechanisms. Clinical and Experimental Pharmacology & Physiology. 1999;**26**(7):493-499

[149] Likar R, Koppert W, Blatnig H, Chiari F, Sittl R, Stein C, et al. Efficacy of peripheral morphine analgesia in inflamed, non-inflamed and perineural tissue of dental surgery patients. Journal of Pain and Symptom Management. 2001;**21**(4):330-337

[150] Stein C. The control of pain in peripheral tissue by opioids. The New England Journal of Medicine. 1995;**332**(25):1685-1690

[151] Stein C. Targeting pain and inflammation by peripherally acting opioids. Frontiers in Pharmacology. 2013;**4**:123

[152] Busch-Dienstfertig M, Stein C. Opioid receptors and opioid peptide-producing leukocytes in inflammatory pain—Basic and therapeutic aspects. Brain, Behavior, and Immunity. 2010;**24**(5):683-694

[153] Stein C, Hassan AH, Lehrberger K, Giefing J, Yassouridis A. Local analgesic effect of endogenous opioid peptides. Lancet. 1993;**342**(8867):321-324

[154] Puehler W, Rittner HL, Mousa SA, Brack A, Krause H, Stein C, et al. Interleukin-1 beta contributes to the upregulation of kappa opioid receptor mrna in dorsal root ganglia in response to peripheral inflammation. Neuroscience. 2006;**141**(2):989-998

[155] Puehler W, Zollner C, Brack A, Shaqura MA, Krause H, Schafer M, et al. Rapid upregulation of mu opioid receptor mRNA in dorsal root ganglia in response to peripheral inflammation depends on neuronal conduction. Neuroscience. 2004;**129**(2):473-479

[156] Hanna MH, Elliott KM, Fung M. Randomized, double-blind study of the analgesic efficacy of morphine-6-glucuronide versus morphine sulfate for postoperative pain in major surgery. Anesthesiology. 2005;**102**(4):815-821

[157] Simonnet G, Rivat C. Opioid-induced hyperalgesia: Abnormal or normal pain? Neuroreport. 2003;**14**(1):1-7

[158] Chu LF, Angst MS, Clark D. Opioid-induced hyperalgesia in humans: Molecular mechanisms and clinical considerations. The Clinical Journal of Pain. 2008;**24**(6):479-496

[159] Roeckel LA, Le Coz GM, Gavériaux Ruff C, Simonin F. Opioid-induced hyperalgesia: Cellular and molecular mechanisms. Neuroscience. 2016;**338**:160-182

[160] Colvin LA, Bull F, Hales TG. Perioperative opioid analgesia—When is

enough too much? A review of opioid-induced tolerance and hyperalgesia. Lancet. 2019;**393**(10180):1558-1568

[161] Corder G, Tawfik VL, Wang D, Sypek EI, Low SA, Dickinson JR, et al. Loss of mu opioid receptor signaling in nociceptors, but not microglia, abrogates morphine tolerance without disrupting analgesia. Nature Medicine. 2017;**23**(2):164-173

[162] Loeza-Alcocer E, McPherson TP, Gold MS. Peripheral GABA receptors regulate colonic afferent excitability and visceral nociception. The Journal of Physiology. 2019;**597**(13):3425-3439

[163] Lotsch J, Weyer-Menkhoff I, Tegeder I. Current evidence of cannabinoid-based analgesia obtained in preclinical and human experimental settings. European Journal of Pain. 2018;**22**(3):471-484

[164] Guo Y, Yao FR, Cao DY, Pickar JG, Zhang Q, Wang HS, et al. Somatostatin inhibits activation of dorsal cutaneous primary afferents induced by antidromic stimulation of primary afferents from an adjacent thoracic segment in the rat. Brain Research. 2008;**1229**:61-71

[165] Wang J, Guo Y, Cao DY, Luo R, Ma SJ, Wang HS, et al. Tonic inhibition of somatostatin on C and Adelta afferent fibers in rat dorsal skin in vivo. Brain Research. 2009;**1288**:50-59

[166] Leppert W, Malec-Milewska M, Zajaczkowska R, Wordliczek J. Transdermal and topical drug administration in the treatment of pain. Molecules. 2018;**23**(3):e23030681

[167] Baron R, Hans G, Dickenson AH. Peripheral input and its importance for central sensitization. Annals of Neurology. 2013;**74**(5):630-636

Chapter 9

Interventional Treatment Options for Trigeminal Neuralgia

Yashar Eshraghi, Sarah J. Vitug and Maged Guirguis

Abstract

Trigeminal neuralgia is characterized by sudden and severe shock-like episodes of transient unilateral pain in the trigeminal nerve distribution. Most cases are idiopathic and are known to respond favorably to anticonvulsants. For patients who fail at least three drug trials or experience intolerable side effects, surgery may be warranted. First, a diagnostic block at the trigeminal nerve or Gasserian ganglion to confirm clinical diagnosis is performed. Surgical intervention can be either ablative or nonablative, each with its respective indications, contraindications, and risk-benefit profile. Most common are the percutaneous rhizotomies: conventional and pulsed radiofrequency ablation (RFA), chemical glycerol injections, and mechanical balloon compression. Stereotactic or gamma knife radiosurgery (GKRS) is the least invasive with only a moderate duration of pain relief, whereas microvascular decompression (VMD) is the most invasive, but associated with greatest long-term benefit. RFA has consistently shown favorable results and is the only modality with evidence of pain relief in ≥50% of patients treated 20 years postoperatively. Auxiliary interventional options such as peripheral neurectomy, botulinum toxin type-A (BTX-A) injections, and cryotherapy are available for those with contraindications to rhizotomies, radiosurgery, or neurosurgery. Ultimately, physicians must tailor their management of trigeminal neuralgia to the needs of the patient.

Keywords: trigeminal neuralgia, Meckel's cave, Gasserian ganglion, ophthalmic division, maxillary division, mandibular division, classic approach, coronoid approach, trigeminal nerve block, Gasserian ganglion block, percutaneous radiofrequency rhizotomy, percutaneous glycerol rhizotomy, percutaneous balloon compression, stereotactic radiosurgery, gamma knife radiosurgery, microvascular decompression, peripheral neurectomy, botulinum toxin type-A, cryotherapy, cryoanalgesia

1. Introduction

Trigeminal neuralgia, also known as "tic douloureux," is characterized by distinctive, transient episodes of unilateral lancinating pain in the trigeminal nerve distribution [1]. Most often, etiology is unknown and is not attributed to another disorder. This presentation is referred to as Type I or classic trigeminal neuralgia. Inflammatory causes (e.g., multiple sclerosis, infection, etc.), compression of the trigeminal roots (e.g., tumors and arteriovenous malformation), abnormalities of the skull base [2], or pain due to underlying disease processes comprise Type II or secondary trigeminal neuralgia. Atypical or mixed trigeminal neuralgia is when patients experience sensory loss or dull, burning pain in the trigeminal nerve distribution in between the characteristic paroxysms [2], and often without an identifiable trigger zone. Atypical disease is more commonly associated with a symptomatic presentation or background pain of milder intensity for up to 50% of the time [3].

Patients usually describe the pain as sudden and severe electric, shooting or shock-like, and superficial pain lasting anywhere from a few seconds to several minutes [2]. Attacks are considered paroxysmal, where frequency of episodes can range from a few to several dozens in 1 day [3]. Additionally, paroxysms are generally similar in nature for individual patients. The pain associated with the classic presentation can be precipitated by light mechanical stimulation to the face or oral mucosa (e.g., facial hair grooming and tooth brushing) or by thermal stimulation (e.g., cold or heat exposure) [2]. It is common for patients to develop an aversion to eating, drinking, or previous noxious stimuli for fear of triggering another episode. More so, the psychological impact may cause patients to appear distressed or anxious during physical examination [4]. For these reasons, the unique presentation with the absence of other neurologic abnormalities makes trigeminal neuralgia a clinical diagnosis [2]. Dental X-rays or MRIs may be warranted to clarify differential diagnoses or confirm a suspected etiology which may guide management.

Overall, trigeminal neuralgia is considered a rare disease according to population-based studies, with estimated 4–13 cases diagnosed per 100,000 individuals each year [5]. However, regional biases exist where countries with less stringent diagnostic criteria yield a higher incidence. For example, the annual incidence of disease in the United Kingdom (26.8 per 100,000 cases) is based off general practitioner lists and fewer diagnostic criteria, compared to the United States (5.9) and Netherlands (12.6), respectively [3].

Anatomically, the vast majority of cases affect either the maxillary or mandibular division (V2 or V3), alone or in combination. In approximately 5% of patients, the symptoms occur solely in the ophthalmic division (V1). In terms of disease onset, trigeminal neuralgia rarely manifests in individuals younger than age 40, with incidence peaking in the elderly and more than twice as many women affected than men [6]. However, it is important to note that trigeminal neuralgia is considered a progressive disease with symptomatic treatment with repeat procedures becoming less effective over time [3].

2. First-line management of medication-resistant trigeminal neuralgia

The primary treatment for trigeminal neuralgia is pharmacologic. Pain associated with trigeminal neuralgia responds poorly to analgesics and favorably to antiepileptic drugs. First-line medical treatment is carbamazepine, with other adjuncts such as phenytoin, gabapentin, lamotrigine, or baclofen added for persistent pain [4].

Patients with intolerable medication side effects or who experience pain refractory to three attempted drug trials and are surgically fit as dictated by medical status/age may be considered for surgery [7]. Patients may first undergo preliminary nerve blocks either at the level of a trigeminal nerve branch or at the Gasserian ganglion to confirm the diagnosis of trigeminal neuralgia. If patients experience pain relief with this diagnostic procedure, patients may elect further therapeutic treatment with the same modality or discuss different surgical treatment options with their neurologist, neurosurgeon, anesthesiologist, or other physicians involved in their care [8].

Surgical methods for the treatment of trigeminal neuralgia can be separated into four broad categories—peripheral lesions to the terminal branches, lesions to the trigeminal (Gasserian) ganglion, lesions to the ganglion root by stereotactic radiosurgery or gamma knife radiosurgery (GKRS), and posterior fossa intervention with microvascular decompression (MVD) [9]. Alternatively, surgical intervention can be divided into non-ablative/nondestructive (MVD) and ablative (all other surgical interventions).

The non-ablative MVD is a complex posterior fossa procedure requiring a craniotomy and thus is performed exclusively by neurosurgeons [10]. This approach is rapidly becoming the surgical intervention of choice when there is MRI-confirmed vascular compression by the nerve root as pain relief is significant, and severe complication risks such as death and relapse rate are among the lowest of all surgical treatment modalities [3]. If no compression is found, percutaneous rhizotomies via thermal (pulsed radiofrequency or thermocoagulation), chemical (glycerol), or mechanical (balloon compression) techniques or gamma knife radiosurgery (GKRS) are preferred. As sensory ablation by rhizotomy demonstrate similar pain relief results in comparison to MVD, it is important for patients to consider the slightly higher risk of complications and slightly lower patient satisfaction at 5-year follow-up with rhizotomies [10]. GKRS is also a safe and effective treatment; however, patients are counseled on the likelihood of a delayed onset of pain relief following treatment, and those with a significant surgical history involving the head may make poor candidates for GKRS [9].

3. Second-line management of medication-resistant trigeminal neuralgia

Ultimately, patient preferences for surgical intervention are always taken into consideration and only if medical status permits. For patients who wish to undergo intervention for management of their medically refractory disease and do not wish to have MVD, any form of rhizotomy, or GKRS, patients may elect to have other treatments such as peripheral neurectomy, botulinum toxin type-A (BTX-A) injections, or cryotherapy. Such interventions can be administered by a variety of physicians such as oral and maxillofacial surgeons, anesthesiologists, neurologists, and other certified providers in both inpatient and outpatient settings.

Peripheral or mental neurectomy under local anesthesia is still offered for management of pharmacologically resistant trigeminal neuralgia; however, it is most often used in rural areas where more advanced surgical options (MVD, rhizotomy, GKRS) are unavailable or unaffordable [11]. Neurectomies essentially are too underreported to gauge its actual utility compared to other treatments. BTX-A is another minimally invasive approach, which can be performed in an outpatient setting and repeated a number of times without significant adverse effects. However, the location (intradermal or intramuscular) and dosage (25–75 units) per injection have yet to be standardized [12]. Anecdotally, cryotherapy is one of the more painful procedures and does not appear to have significant long-term efficacy in pain relief compared to other interventions. It is maintained that cryogenic insult varies with nerve diameter and is thus associated with variable nerve regeneration and shorter pain-free intervals [13].

Often, patients electing these auxiliary interventions have major contraindications for neurosurgery, are unfit for general anesthesia, or simply prefer less invasive procedures [14–16]. However, the effectiveness, duration of pain relief, rate of relapse and complication, and overall patient satisfaction with auxiliary interventions are generally based on case reports and studies with small sample sizes; thus, overall impression of such modalities is less favorable compared to MVD, rhizotomy, and GKRS [17].

4. Complications

As with any invasive procedure, patients must be counseled on postoperative risk for infection and bleeding (hematomas) at the site of needle entry or incision. With trigeminal nerve and Gasserian ganglion blocks, a small risk of dysesthesias or a loss of consciousness may occur if CSF is inadvertently injected with local anesthetic [8]. For patients undergoing MVD, rhizotomy procedures, or GKRS, postoperative hyperesthesia, facial asymmetry, masseter weakness, alteration in corneal sensation, and meningitis are extremely rare complications; however, patients must always be informed of potential risks [8]. As with the auxiliary intervention options, patients are educated on the similar complications such as dysesthesias, facial weakness, and asymmetry, albeit rare. Of note, cryotherapy is one technique that attempts to preserve sensation post-procedure.

5. Conclusion

It is imperative that patients accurately assess pain levels before and after surgical intervention to better guide treatment options in the future if relapse occurs. Patients must understand that most of these surgical interventions may not rid their symptoms of trigeminal neuralgia permanently and that large, randomized controlled trials are needed to thoroughly predict the long-term efficacy of these interventions and disease prognosis. The paucity of standardization in the follow-up period for patients undergoing surgical treatment is generally physician-specific and on a case-by-case basis, depending on the severity of disease and wishes of the patient. However, the consensus in the literature is that surgical management for the treatment of medication-refractory trigeminal neuralgia is safe and effective.

5.1 Trigeminal (Gasserian) ganglion, maxillary nerve, and mandibular nerve blocks

Gasserian ganglion, maxillary nerve, and mandibular nerve blocks play an integral role as a diagnostic block prior to trigeminal neurolysis, if indicated.

Patients who report significant pain reduction (greater than 50% compared to preoperative baseline) from two consecutive diagnostic blocks are recommended subsequent percutaneous procedures for a more sustained therapeutic effect.

5.2 Gasserian ganglion nerve block

5.2.1 Anatomy

The trigeminal nerve contains sensory and motor fibers. Somatic afferent fibers transmit pain, light touch, and temperature sensation from the skin of the face, the oral and nasal mucosa, the teeth, and the anterior two thirds of the tongue. Visceral efferent fibers innervate muscles of facial expression, the tensor tympani, and muscles of mastication. Also, the trigeminal nerve has multiple communications with autonomic nervous system through the ciliary, sphenopalatine, and optic and submaxillary ganglia.

The trigeminal nerve travels as follows: brain stem, prepontine fossa, Meckel's cave (trigeminal/Gasserian ganglion location), and extracranial. The ganglion (approximately 1 × 2 cm) can be found within a reflection of dura mater known as Meckel's cave, which lies in the middle cranial fossa adjacent to the petrous bone. Superior to Meckel's cave is the inferior surface of the temporal lobe, posterior is the brain stem, and medial is the cavernous sinus and internal carotid artery. After the Gasserian ganglion, the nerve separates somatotopically into the following divisions: ophthalmic (craniomedially), mandibular (caudolaterally), and maxillary in between [8].

Indications:

- Diagnostic block to confirm clinical diagnosis of trigeminal neuralgia [8]
- Therapeutic block in medically refractory cases
- Prognostic indicator for planned neuroablative or surgical procedure
- Diagnosis and management of various orofacial pain syndromes (e.g., cluster headache, persistent ocular pain, palliation of cancer pain)

Contraindications: the contraindications to Gasserian ganglion nerve block are the same as those for trigeminal nerve block: patient refusal, local infection, sepsis, coagulopathy, increased intracranial pressure, behavioral abnormalities, allergy to local anesthetics, and lack of patient cooperation.

Approach: the patient is positioned supine with the cervical spine extended. As the patient's cooperation is paramount, the procedure is usually done under local anesthetic and sedation [18]. Under fluoroscopic guidance, submental (**Figure 1a**) and lateral (**Figure 1b**) views are obtained to identify the foramen ovale [18]. Approximately 2.5 cm lateral to the corner of the mouth, a needle is advanced perpendicular to the pupil of the eye in a cephalad direction toward the auditory meatus. Once the needle tip has made contact with the base of the skull, the needle is withdrawn slightly and walked posteriorly into the foramen ovale. The needle is carefully aspirated to confirm the absence of CSF/blood prior to therapeutic

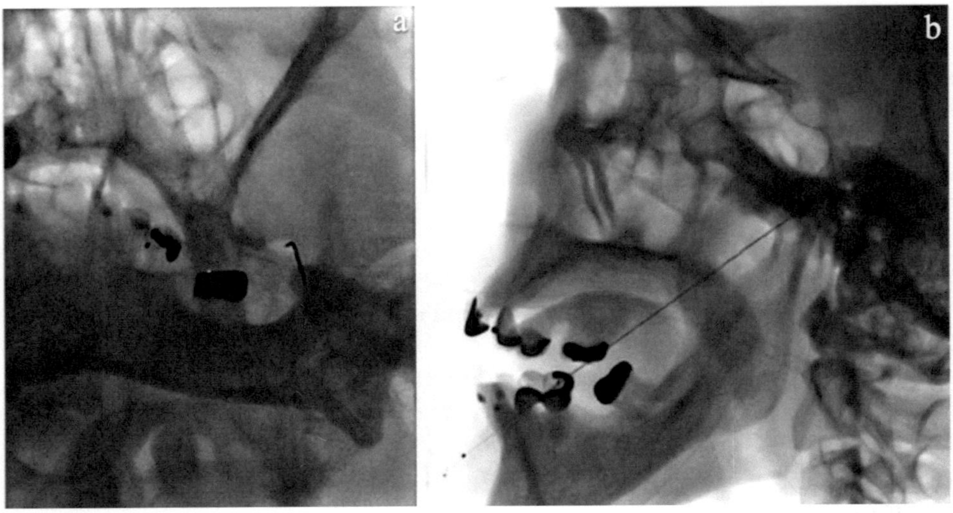

Figure 1.
Submental (a) and lateral (b) view of needle in foramen ovale [18].

injection. After needle position is confirmed and aspiration is negative, an average volume of 0.4 mL of neurolytic solution is injected.

Complications: due to the close relation between the Gasserian ganglion and the dural reflection, Meckel's cave, inadvertent local anesthetic injection into CSF causing loss of consciousness is a feared complication of this procedure [19]. Additionally, dysesthesias [17] and hematoma formation upon needle entry into the foramen ovale are other complications associated with this technique.

Outcome: the overall therapeutic benefit of the Gasserian ganglion block is largely similar to that of trigeminal nerve block, with most patients reporting pain relief greater than 50% of baseline for up to 6–12 months [18] and much shorter duration if used as a diagnostic block.

5.3 Maxillary nerve and mandibular nerve blocks

5.3.1 Anatomy

The maxillary division (V2) is the second division of the trigeminal nerve, which exits the middle cranial fossa through the foramen rotundum, located at the roof of the pterygopalatine fossa (PPF) [8]. V2 provides purely sensory fibers to the lower eyelid, cheek, nares, upper lip, upper teeth, upper gums, nasal mucosa, palate, roof of the pharynx, maxillary sinus, ethmoid sinus, sphenoid sinus, and parts of the meninges.

Its branches are divided into four groups, depending on the location where they branch off: the cranium, the pterygopalatine fossa, the infraorbital canal, or the face [20]. The intracranial group includes the middle meningeal nerve [20]. The pterygopalatine group includes the zygomatic nerve, the superior alveolar nerves, the nasopalatine nerve, the palatine nerves, and the pharyngeal nerve [21]. The infraorbital group includes the infraorbital nerve and the anterior superior alveolar nerve [8]. The facial group includes the inferior palpebral nerve, the superior labial nerve, and the lateral nasal nerve.

The mandibular division (V3) is the third division of the trigeminal nerve, which exits the middle cranial fossa via the foramen ovale (≤1 cm in diameter), situated immediately dorsolateral to the pterygoid process [19]. V3 contains a large sensory root and a small motor root that provide innervation to the lower lip, lower teeth, gums, chin, jaw, parts of the external ear, and parts of the meninges. However, the mandibular division is known for providing motor innervation to the muscles of mastication.

Its branches are divided into three groups: the main trunk, the anterior division, and the posterior division [20]. The main trunk group includes efferent branches for the medial pterygoid, tensor tympani, tensor veli palatini muscles, and an afferent nerve for the meningeal branch [20]. The anterior group includes the efferent masseteric, deep temporal, and lateral pterygoid nerves and the afferent buccal nerve [21]. The posterior group includes the efferent/afferent inferior alveolar nerve and the afferent auriculotemporal and lingual nerves.

Indications:

- Diagnostic block in assessment and management of trigeminal neuralgia and atypical facial pain [8]
- Anatomic differential neural blockade when more selective nerve block needed for diagnosis of various orofacial pain syndromes
- Therapeutic block for acute pain emergencies [18]
- Diagnosis and management of various orofacial pain syndromes (e.g., cluster headache, persistent ocular pain, palliation of cancer pain)

Contraindications: the contraindications for performing maxillary and mandibular nerve blocks include but are not limited to the following: patient refusal, local infection, sepsis, coagulopathy, increased intracranial pressure, behavioral abnormalities, allergy to local anesthetics, and lack of patient cooperation.

Approach: patients are placed supine with cervical spine extended. The anesthesiologist should be at the patient's side, approximately shoulder level. The site of needle puncture is medial to the masseter muscle (~3 cm lateral to the corner of the mouth) which can be identified by asking the patient to clench his or her teeth. Following the initial numbing, evidenced by the raised skin wheal, a 22-gauge, 10-cm needle is inserted with fluoroscopic guidance [19]. Needle insertion is aligned with the pupil to a depth of 4.5–6 cm to contact the infratemporal surface of the greater wing of the sphenoid, immediately anterior to the foramen ovale [19]. The needle is then retracted and advanced into the foramen ovale to a final depth of 6–7 cm, often resulting in mandibular paresthesia, followed by paresthesia in the ophthalmic and maxillary nerve distribution with further needle advancement. Injection of contrast will identify vascular uptake and extent of injectate spread [22]. Prior to injection with local anesthetic, the needle should be carefully aspirated to confirm the absence of CSF/blood. One millimeter of local anesthetic is generally adequate for a diagnostic nerve block to occur within 5–10 minutes.

The coronoid approach may be utilized for selective maxillary and mandibular nerve block. The coronoid notch is identified by asking the patient to open and close the mouth several times and palpating the area just anterior and slightly inferior to the acoustic auditory meatus. A needle is inserted just below the zygomatic arch directly in the middle of the coronoid notch and placement verified on lateral view (**Figure 2a**). The needle is advanced 2.5–5 cm in a plane perpendicular to the skull until the lateral pterygoid plate is encountered. Needle placement is verified on PA view (**Figure 2b**). Injection of contrast will identify vascular uptake and extent of injectate spread. The needle is withdrawn slightly, and an incremental injection technique of 3–5 mL of local anesthetic is administered to each nerve [22].

Complications: hematoma formation upon needle entry into the foramen ovale and local anesthetic toxicity are the major complications associated with this procedure [22]. However, dysesthesias, weakness of the muscles of mastication, secondary facial asymmetry, meningitis, intracranial hemorrhage with inadvertent intracranial needle placement, total spinal anesthesia, and anesthesia dolorosa are other complications associated with trigeminal nerve blocks [22].

Outcome: as a therapeutic block, effects of trigeminal nerve block are relatively short term, with most patients reporting pain relief greater than 50% of baseline for up to 6–12 months [18]. However, as trigeminal nerve blocks are primarily diagnostic, short-term pain relief is expected.

5.4 Interventional treatment for trigeminal neuralgia: percutaneous rhizotomies and neuromodulation

Peripheral lesions to the terminal branches with therapeutic intent are usually via radiofrequency thermocoagulation or highly concentrated alcohol injections [9] and less commonly with neurectomy, Botox injections, or cryolesions; however, adequate trials supporting these modalities are yet to surface [17].

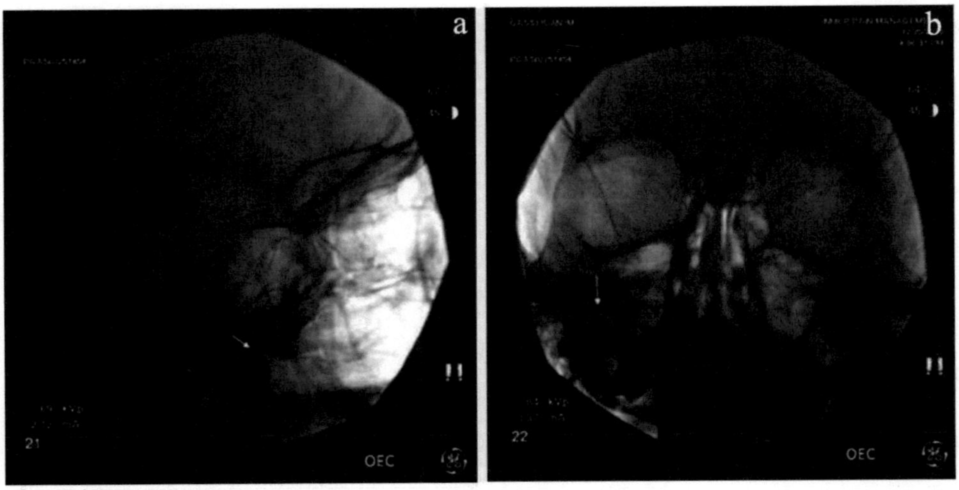

Figure 2.
Lateral view (a): needle inserted (white arrow) coaxially in coronoid notch. PA view (b): needle (white arrow) advanced medially until contact is made with lateral pterygoid plate [22].

Percutaneous lesions to the Gasserian ganglion are traditionally in the form of rhizotomies, radiofrequency, and chemical lesions by glycerol, phenol, or alcohol injection [18] but also via mechanical compression from balloon inflation. Ganglion-level procedures are generally preferred as they are safer and more effective than peripheral techniques [23], as all procedures are carried out under fluoroscopic guidance [9].

5.4.1 Percutaneous radiofrequency rhizotomy (PRR): pulsed radiofrequency ablation and radiofrequency thermocoagulation

Indications:

- Treatment of trigeminal neuralgia in a medically refractory or side-effect-intolerable patient

- High-risk operative patients such as the medically ill or elderly [24]

- Secondary trigeminal neuralgia due to multiple sclerosis [25]

- Diagnostic procedure in patients with atypical disease (constant or near constant pain in addition to the classic sharp stabbing pains in trigeminal nerve distribution) [26]

- Patient preference for minimally invasive procedure

Contraindications: contraindications for PRR are patient refusal, local infection, sepsis, coagulopathy, increased intracranial pressure, behavioral abnormalities, allergy to local anesthetics, and lack of patient cooperation. Radiofrequency thermocoagulation may be contraindicated in postherpetic neuralgia [25].

Approach: the patient is placed supine with cervical spine slightly extended. Procedure requires patient cooperation; thus, it is performed under local anesthetic and light sedation [18]. Under C-arm fluoroscopic guidance, a needle is introduced 2.5 cm lateral to the corner of the mouth. Advancement of the needle medial to the ramus of the jaw into the foramen ovale is verified on oblique view (**Figure 3a**). The use of bony landmarks and fluoroscopic guidance facilitates accurate radiofrequency needle placement to locate Meckel's cave through the foramen ovale. Needle placement is confirmed with lateral fluoroscopic view (**Figure 3b**) prior to neurolysis [24].

Through stepwise advancement of the needle toward the Gasserian ganglion, V3 is first encountered, followed by V2 and lastly V1 [26]. Once in Meckel's cave, aspiration may yield CSF. The stylet is then replaced with the electrode to confirm that nerve root stimulation coincides with location of paresthesia felt by patient. Following accurate needle placement, the patient is anesthetized prior to thermal lesioning in cycles of 45–90 seconds at temperatures between 60 and 90°C [26]. Other parameters have utilized 60-second cycles at 70°C [8]. Pulsed radiofrequency is set to 42°C for 120-second cycles. Patient is awakened in between cycles for manual sensory testing throughout the face until complete pain resolution has been achieved.

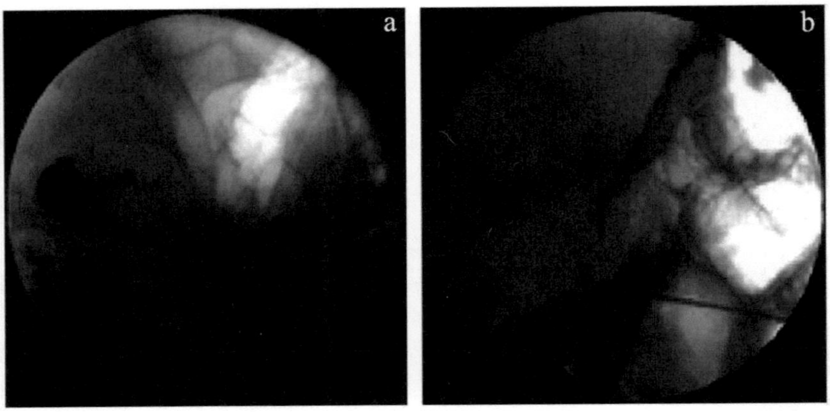

Figure 3.
Oblique view (a) verifies needle placement medial to the ramus of the jaw prior to entry into the foramen ovale. Lateral view (b) confirms needle position prior to injuring the trigeminal nerve, a technique used with PRR, percutaneous glycerol rhizotomy (PGR), or percutaneous balloon compression (PBC) [24].

Complications: complications associated with PRR are decreased corneal sensation with increased risk of keratitis, masseter weakness, hyperesthesia, and although very rare, anesthesia dolorosa.

Outcome: pain relief immediately following procedure is very high, with 97.6–99% of patients reporting full resolution. Pain relief was reported to be 61.8% at 1 year, 57.7% at 5 years, 52.3% at 10 years, and 41% at 20 years. PRR appears to be the only surgical intervention with long-term follow-up at 20 years [24].

5.4.2 Percutaneous glycerol rhizotomy (PGR)

Indications:

- Treatment of trigeminal neuralgia in a medically refractory or side-effect-intolerable patient and other high-risk operative patients such as the medically ill or elderly [24]

- Patients who have previously undergone MVD or have history of multiple sclerosis [27]

- Diagnostic procedure in patients with atypical disease (constant or near constant pain in addition to the classic sharp, stabbing pains in trigeminal nerve distribution) [26]

- Patient preference for a minimally invasive procedure

Contraindications: contraindications to PGR are patient refusal, local infection, sepsis, coagulopathy, increased intracranial pressure, behavioral abnormalities, allergy to local anesthetics, and lack of patient cooperation.

Approach: the patient is placed supine with the cervical spine slightly extended. Percutaneous techniques require patient cooperation during intermittent anesthetization; thus, procedures are performed under local anesthetic and sedation [18]. Under C-arm fluoroscopic imaging, a needle is introduced

2.5 cm lateral to the corner of the mouth. The needle is inserted into the trigeminal cistern through the foramen ovale. Precise needle placement must be ascertained prior to puncture as subarachnoid entry beneath the temporal lobe may yield significant complications. CSF may be encountered when the needle contacts the Gasserian ganglion, unless patient has previously received surgical intervention in this area [26]. Radiopaque contrast is then utilized to visualize the cistern prior to glycerol gangliolysis. Patient is repositioned to a sitting position for a test dose of sterile anhydrous glycerol, followed by dose escalation of 0.1–0.4 mL total. Patient must remain seated for approximately 2 hours postinjection [26].

Complications: complications associated with PGR are hyperesthesia, decreased corneal sensation, facial hematoma, aseptic meningitis, hearing loss, bacterial meningitis, buccal mucosa penetration, and carotid puncture.

Outcome: pain relief immediately following PGR is good, however, still below that from PRR and with greater variability; 71–97.9% of patients report full resolution immediately following procedure. Pain relief was reported to be between 53 and 63% at 1 year and 43.5% at 5 years [24]. No further time points have been collected for PGR.

5.4.3 Percutaneous balloon compression (PBC)

Indications:

- Treatment of trigeminal neuralgia in a medically refractory or side-effect-intolerable patient and other high-risk operative patients such as the medically ill or elderly [24]

- Diagnostic procedure in patients with atypical disease (constant or near constant pain in addition to the classic sharp, stabbing pains in trigeminal nerve distribution) [26]

- Patient preference for minimally invasive procedure

Contraindications: PBC may be relatively contraindicated in patients with underlying cardiac disease as trigeminal reflex bradycardia and hypotension may occur [28].

Approach: the patient is placed in a supine position with the neck and thorax slightly extended 29]. However, another approach involves the patient semi-seated with head retroflexed to obtain a submental vertical X-ray beam for a horizontal view of the foramen ovale [30]. Patient undergoes endotracheal intubation and general anesthesia. C-arm fluoroscopy is used for anteroposterior and lateral images to confirm needle placement. A 14-gauge needle is inserted approximately 2.5 cm lateral to the corner of the mouth, parallel to the sagittal plane to protect the oral mucosa. Under fluoroscopic guidance, the catheter is redirected to the foramen ovale. A no. 4 Fogarty catheter is then advanced to 10–15 mm beyond the needle tip. The balloon is inflated until proximal to the posterior fossa with approximately 300 mg of I_2/mL iohexol [29]. Compression volume is patient specific, until pear-shaped balloon is achieved with respect to the nearby structures (e.g., clivus, sella, and petrous bones). The contrast medium is aspirated, catheter is withdrawn, and pressure is applied to needle entry site.

Complications: complications associated with PBC are hyperesthesia with persistent symptoms, masseter weakness, facial hematoma, hearing loss, anesthesia dolorosa, decreased corneal sensation, pseudoaneurysm, bacterial meningitis, septic meningitis, trigeminal reflex bradycardia, and hypotension.

Outcome: pain relief immediately following PBC is also promising, however, still below that from PRR; 82–93.8% of patients report full resolution immediately following procedure. Pain relief was reported to be between 74.6% at 1 year, 69.8% at 5 years, and between 30 and 51.5% at 10 years [24]. No further time points have been collected for PBC.

5.4.4 Stereotactic radiosurgery/gamma knife radiosurgery (GKRS)

Indications:

- Patients who are surgically unfit for MVD due to significant medical comorbidities
- Patients who refuse to take anticonvulsants
- Patients currently on anticoagulation therapy [31]

Contraindications: as this noninvasive outpatient procedure is considered one of the safest surgical techniques in the treatment of trigeminal neuralgia, few contraindications have been reported. Patients who have had an extensive history of surgical intervention may be at an increased risk of complications [24].

Approach: the patient is supine with mild oral or intravenous sedation. A Leksell Model G stereotactic frame is secured to the patient's head with local anesthetic [26]. MRI maps the neurovascular compression at the entry zone of the trigeminal nerve. Once exact intracranial location is confirmed, a 4-mm collimator is used, with radiation dose prescribed to 100% isodose line [32]. The isocenter is placed near the pars triangularis and highly focused beams of radiation (70–90 Gy) to the trigeminal nerve root in the posterior fossa [7].

Complications: complications of GKRS are dose dependent, with increased rate of occurrence rate with cumulative radiation dose exceeding 115 Gy. Alternatively, the rate of complications increases when GKRS is performed following failed treatment with other surgical interventions [24]. Hyperesthesias were reported in 6–42% of patients, and anesthesia dolorosa occurred at a rate of 0.2% [33].

Outcome: pain relief associated with GKRS can be delayed up to 8 weeks [9] postoperatively (mean time of 1 month) and is highly dependent on the accuracy of the stereotactic system used [7]. Between 79 and 91.8% of individuals had pain relief; however, a mean delay of 10 days to 3.4 months was experienced prior to initial pain relief. Further follow-ups identified 75–90% of patients with pain relief at 1 year, 44–65% at 5 years, and 30–51.5% of individuals with pain relief at 10 years.

5.4.5 Microvascular decompression (MVD)

Indications:

- Medically refractory patients who are deemed surgically fit as by medical status/age [7]

- First-line treatment in younger patients due to long-term improvement in quality of life [34]

Contraindications: although advanced age is a relative contraindication, there is no age limit for this procedure as long as patients are fit to undergo general anesthesia [26].

Approach: the patient is placed in a lateral decubitus position, which allows for easier lumbar puncture and CSF drainage to decrease tension in infratentorial space. A suboccipital craniotomy is performed to enter the posterior fossa, targeting the trigeminal nerve-pons junction [26]. The infratentorial lateral supracerebellar approach accesses the trigeminal nerve within the superior portion of the cerebellopontine angle via the lateral aspect of the cerebellar tentorial surface [35]. Once the CSF is aspirated, retraction of the superolateral margin of the cerebellum facilitates contact with the nerve. Most commonly, the superior cerebellar artery (SCA) is responsible for nerve compression at the root entry zone and, less commonly, the anterior inferior cerebellar artery or superior petrosal veins [36]. Thus, the arachnoid membrane must be dissected from the trigeminal nerve all throughout its course through Meckel's cavity in order to expose the compression. The SCA courses medial to the trigeminal nerve, which always compresses the nerve medially. Retraction of the cerebellum should be minimized as injury to the vestibulocochlear nerve is at risk. For transposition of the compressing artery, the sling retraction technique is used [37].

Complications: complications associated with MVD are trigeminal nerve deficit, facial weakness, hearing loss, anesthesia dolorosa, aseptic meningitis, hydrocephalus, mortality, and cerebellar infarct or hematoma [24].

Outcome: long-term pain relief from MVD has been found to be superior among existing surgical interventions for treatment of trigeminal neuralgia at this time; thus, it is generally considered to be first-line intervention for operative candidates [24]. Between 80.3 and 96% of patients experienced initial pain relief immediately following MVD, 84% at 1 year, 72–85% at 5 years, and 74% at 10 years [24] (**Tables 1** and **2**).

5.5 Other treatment options for trigeminal neuralgia

5.5.1 Peripheral neurectomy

Indications:

- Medically refractory trigeminal neuralgia in patients who are unable to undergo general anesthesia (frail, elderly, or medically unstable patients), as this can be performed as an outpatient procedure under local anesthesia [11]
- Therapeutic for patients reluctant to undergo major neurosurgery or have contraindications for craniotomy when rhizotomies are not possible [49]
- Rural settings where too large surgical facilities may be inaccessible

Contraindications: peripheral neurectomy may be contraindicated in those unable to tolerate general anesthesia, as other approaches are more invasive (e.g., maxillary sinus route) [49].

Summary of complications		
Procedure	**Complication**	**Rate (%)**
PRR	Decreased corneal sensation; keratitis	5.7–17.3; 0.6–1.9 [38]
	Masseter weakness	4 [39]
	Hyperesthesia	3.3 [40]
	Anesthesia dolorosa	0.6–0.8 [39]
PGR	Hyperesthesia	23.3–72 [41]
	Decreased corneal sensation	6.3–15 [40]
	Facial hematoma	7 [42]
	Aseptic meningitis	0.12–3 [42]
	Hearing loss	1.9 [42]
	Bacterial meningitis	1.5–1.7 [42]
	Buccal mucosa penetration	1.5 [42]
	Carotid puncture	0.77 [42]
PBC	Hyperesthesia; persistent symptoms	89–100; 4.6–40 [41]
	Masseter weakness	1.2–12 [39]
	Facial hematoma	3.5–6.7 [43]
	Hearing loss	2.4–6.3 [44]
	Anesthesia dolorosa	0–3.4 [39]
	Decreased corneal sensation	0–3.1 [40]
	Pseudoaneurysm	1 [44]
	Bacterial meningitis	0.7–1 [43]
	Aseptic meningitis	0.7 [43]
	Trigeminal reflex bradycardia	
	Hypotension	
GKRS	Hyperesthesia	6–42 [33]
	Anesthesia dolorosa	0.2 [33]
MVD	Trigeminal nerve deficit	1.6–22 [45]
	Facial weakness	0.6–10.6 [45]
	Hearing loss	1.2–6.8 [45]
	Anesthesia dolorosa	0–4 [46]
	Aseptic meningitis	2 [47]
	Hydrocephalus	0.15 [48]
	Mortality	0.15–0.8 [24]
	Cerebellar infarct or hematoma	0.075–0.68 [45]

Table 1.
Summary of complications and rates associated with PRR, PGR, PBC, GKRS, and MVD [24].

Summary of outcomes					
Procedure	**Initial response (%) rate**	**1-year**	**5-year**	**10-year**	**20-year**
PRR	97.6–99	61.8	57.7	52.3	41
PGR	71–97.9	53–63	43.5		
PBC	82–93.8	74.6	69.8	30–51.5	
GKRS	79–91.8 (Delayed 10 days–3.4 months)	75–90	44–65	30–51.5	
MVD	80.3–96	84	72–85	74	

Table 2.
Summary of success rates of PRR, PGR, PBC, GKRS, and MVD immediately following procedure, 1-, 5-, 10-, and 20-year time points [24].

Approach: for procedures done under local anesthesia, a diagnostic nerve block with 2% lidocaine HCl plus adrenaline 1:200,000 concentration must completely resolve symptoms prior to neurectomy [14]. Infraorbital, inferior alveolar, and mental neurectomies usually require the following incisions: vestibular, Ginwalla's, and crevicular incision, respectively. Clamping and avulsion of the mental nerve require an additional Y-shaped incision along the anterior border of the ascending ramus. After further blunt and sharp dissection on its medial aspect, the temporalis and medial pterygoid muscles are split, facilitating the clamping and avulsing of the mental nerve at the mental foramen. Sealing the infraorbital foramen with stainless steel screws is the final step [14].

For procedures done under general anesthesia, patients are supine, and an intra-oral mucoperiosteal incision is made between the buccal sulcus of the upper lateral incisor to the first molar on the symptomatic side [49]. Once the infraorbital fossa is exposed, access to the maxillary sinus is gained via bone window with a diameter of 2 cm in the anterior wall of the maxillary sinus. Further dissection completely liberates the entire neurovascular bundle in the maxillary sinus, and the removal of the inferior bone of the infraorbital canal and fissure ensues [49]. Another round bone window with 1.5 cm diameter is made at the upper 1/3 of the posterior wall of the maxillary sinus with extreme care as injury to the maxillary artery may occur. The superior bony wall of the maxillary sinus is removed to expose the pterygopalatine fossa segment of the maxillary nerve. The length of the maxillary nerve from the infraorbital foramen to the pterygopalatine fossa is removed, along with the branches of the infraorbital nerve [49].

Complications: anesthesia or paresthesia in the maxillary distribution post-operatively is common and short-lasting. The major complications regarding the pterygoid palatine fossa segment neurectomy of the maxillary nerve under general anesthesia are bleeding, infection, and eye or encephalic injuries.

Outcome: pain relief from peripheral neurectomies has been reported to an average of 26.5 months when obturated with fatty tissues [50] and greater than 24 months when obturated with stainless steel screws [14]. One case report from India of a 65-year-old female who underwent a mental neurectomy endorsed pain reduction from 8 to 1 on VAS score from pre-procedure to 2 years postoperatively, respectively [11]. In terms of recurrence rate, a Danish study evaluated patients at a mean follow-up time of 7 years and reported 78% of patients experienced a recurrence, with half of this group becoming symptomatic within the first month [51]. A study that evaluated 40 patients treated with neurectomy, of whom 28 had previously undergone radiofrequency lesions, 5 of these patients had recurrence after 2 years and were successfully treated with repeat neurectomy [52]. Thus, it can be inferred that mean follow-up time for neurectomy patients in the setting of trigeminal neuralgia is incredibly variable, with sparse reliable data to support findings.

5.5.2 Botulinum toxin type-A (BTX-A) injections

Indications:

- Medically refractory trigeminal neuralgia in patients who desire minimally invasive procedures or are unable to general anesthesia (frail, elderly, or medically unstable patients)

- Patients with contraindications to major neurosurgery

- Patient preference for minimally invasive procedure, as this can be performed outpatient without anesthesia [12]

Contraindications: patients with pre-existing disease that may be exacerbated by exposure to BTX-A (e.g., myasthenia gravis, motor neuron disease, or Lambert-Eaton syndrome), superficial skin infection on treatment site, or the use of drug within 7 days of BTX-A injection that may adversely affect neuromuscular junction (e.g., quinine, aminoglycosides, and penicillamine) [12].

Approach: the number of units and sites to be injected varies per patient. One study approach used a 0.5-mL syringe with 5-/16-inch, 30-gauge needle for subcutaneous injection [53]. Other studies describe injection of unstandardized dosages intramuscularly in the region of the zygomatic arch or masseter [54]. A randomized, double-blind study showed no difference between 25 and 75 units, as both had sustained pain relief at 8 weeks postinjection [12]. Whereas, doses as large as 60 and 40 units of BTX-A diluted in 2.5-mL saline, administered to the external nasal trigger zone and right mental nerve region, respectively, showed sustained relief at 5 months [55].

Complications: as BTX-A injections are generally considered safe; few complications such as short-term (<6 weeks) asymmetry in the injection area during dynamic movement and transient facial edema (<5 days) have been noted [12]. In patients currently on a pharmacologic regimen for trigeminal neuralgia (either analgesic or prophylactic), no adverse effects were noted when combined with BTX-A injections [53].

Outcome: adequate pain control in patients treated with BTX-A has varied between 90 days [15] and 5 months [55]; however, results are largely based on case reports or studies with small sample size. One small, randomized, open-ended study with eight participants underwent BTX-A injections for intractable trigeminal neuralgia found a mean baseline pain score of 4 on VAS, which was reduced to 1.19 at 6 months following treatment [54]. Another study with 13 patients treated with BTX-A and followed at 10-, 20-, 30-, and 60-day postinjection reported pain relief and reduced need for pharmacotherapy in all patients over the course of their study [53]. However, this is often the case where follow-up periods in patients treated with BTX-A and other surgical interventions for their trigeminal neuralgia are not long enough to reliably deduce long-term efficacy.

5.5.3 Cryotherapy (cryoanalgesia)

Indications:

- Medically refractory disease in patients limited to the supraorbital, infraorbital, and mental nerves and potentially the long buccal and lingual nerves
- Elderly or medically compromised patients who are unfit for surgery
- Patient preference for minimally invasive procedure [16]

Contraindications: negligible contraindications have been reported.

Approach: involved nerve branches are identified with test doses of local anesthesia. Upon complete pain abolition, cryotherapy blockades can proceed in an outpatient setting under local anesthesia and intravenous sedation [56].

The approach to the inferior dental nerve cryoblockade utilizes C-arm radiographic guidance, image intensifier, and nerve stimulator on the cryoprobe. Lateral oblique films confirm accurate needle placement prior to alcohol injection around the inferior dental nerve [16].

The approach of cryoblockade to other nerves such as the infraorbital, mental, and inferior alveolar nerves begins with the following incisions: intraoral Caldwell-Luc, intraoral low buccal in the premolar region, and intraoral Ginwalla, respectively. Exposed nerves are frozen with nitrous oxide via cryoprobe at a temperature of −700°C for 2-minute freezing cycles followed by 5 minutes of thawing. This is repeated three times [57].

Complications: potential complications associated with cryoblockade are infection, swelling, trismus, and paresthesia ranging from complete numbness or altered sensation, up to 3 months postoperatively [56]. In a study with 145 patients treated with cryotherapy, 58 patients experienced symptoms of atypical facial pain (symptoms described as burning, pins and needles, or dull ache) which responded to a short course of tricyclic antidepressants [58].

Outcome: duration of pain relief ranges from 6 [56] to 20 months, depending on the treated nerve. A study that looked at 145 patients with paroxysmal trigeminal neuralgia treated with cryotherapy demonstrated a mean relief period of 13 months for long buccal nerve, 17 months for mental, and 20 months for infraorbital nerves [58]. Although well tolerated by patients, multiple sessions of cryotherapy may be needed to achieve durable pain relief, due to regenerative capacity of nerves, albeit subsequent injections are rarely as effective as the first [58]. In a study that looked at 145 patients treated by cryotherapy, 56% of patients needed more than 1 treatment, with a number of patients needing up to 11 procedures. Of the 145 patients, pain relief at 6 months was achieved in half of the group, with only 27% pain-free at 1 year [58].

6. Conclusion

As medical treatment with anticonvulsants has been the cornerstone of first-line management of trigeminal neuralgia, surgical interventions have been developed for more involved cases. Patients who continue to experience pain with three failed drug trials or encounter an intolerable side-effect profile from medications are generally considered for surgical evaluation. However, only patients who are deemed surgically fit per medical status/age shall be recommended for operative procedures.

Diagnostic blocks are fundamental in the surgical evaluation of a patient with medically refractory trigeminal neuralgia. Trigeminal nerve and Gasserian ganglion blocks confirm the clinical diagnosis before the patient can be considered for subsequent intervention. Additional nerve blocks administered to a terminal branch of the trigeminal nerve or at the Gasserian ganglion with therapeutic intent may offer adequate pain control for some patients. Most commonly, patients are treated with percutaneous rhizotomies (radiofrequency, glycerol, and balloon compression), stereotactic radiosurgery, and microvascular decompression for more sustained pain relief with minimal postoperative complications. Other procedures that have fallen out of favor but are still used are peripheral neurectomy include botulinum toxin type-A injections and cryotherapy on a case-by-case basis. It is thought that patients opting for modalities targeting peripheral branches of the trigeminal nerve, rather than the ganglion or nerve root, are more likely to become symptomatic as pain may break through in other nerves not previously treated [59].

Ultimately, all surgical candidates are thoroughly counseled on available interventions and their individual risk-benefit profiles before undergoing further treatment. As all surgical techniques have demonstrated efficacy in the treatment of medically refractory trigeminal neuralgia, patient input on procedure invasiveness, repeatability, accessibility, and cost are all important factors to consider in choosing a treatment. More studies with larger sample size, randomized controlled design, and stricter diagnostic criteria for patients are needed to reliably comment on the prognostic value of each of the aforementioned treatment options. Regardless, it is with a patient-centric, multidisciplinary approach from all physicians involved in a patient's care that the best treatment plan can be implemented for those with intractable trigeminal neuralgia.

Author details

Yashar Eshraghi*, Sarah J. Vitug and Maged Guirguis
Department of Anesthesiology and Critical Care, Ochsner Health System University of Queensland School of Medicine, Australia

*Address all correspondence to: yashar.eshraghi@gmail.com

References

[1] Zakrzewska JM, McMillan R. Trigeminal neuralgia: The diagnosis and management of this excruciating and poorly understood facial pain. Postgraduate Medical Journal. 2011;**87**(1028):410-416

[2] Bennetto L, Patel NK, Fuller G. Trigeminal neuralgia and its management. BMJ. 2007;**334**(7586):201-205

[3] Zakrzewska JM, Linskey ME. Trigeminal neuralgia. BMJ Clinical Evidence. 2014;**2014**:1207

[4] Fields HL. Treatment of trigeminal neuralgia. The New England Journal of Medicine. 1996;**334**(17):1125-1126

[5] MacDonald BK, Cockerell OC, Sander JW, Shorvon SD. The incidence and lifetime prevalence of neurological disorders in a prospective community-based study in the UK. Brain. 2000;**123**(Pt 4):665-676

[6] Katusic S, Beard CM, Bergstralh E, Kurland LT. Incidence and clinical features of trigeminal neuralgia, Rochester, Minnesota, 1945-1984. Annals of Neurology. 1990;**27**(1):89-95

[7] Al-Quliti KW. Update on neuropathic pain treatment for trigeminal neuralgia. The pharmacological and surgical options. Neurosciences (Riyadh). 2015;**20**(2):107-114

[8] Narouze SN. Interventional Management of Head and Face Pain: Nerve Blocks and Beyond. New York, NY: Springer; 2014

[9] Cruccu G. Trigeminal neuralgia. Continuum (Minneap Minn). 2017;**23**(2):396-420

[10] Zakrzewska JM. Surgery for trigeminal neuralgia? Pain. 2011;**152**(3):469-470

[11] Sikkerimath BC, Merchant MI, Patil NS, Mathivanan SM. Peripheral neurectomy for trigeminal neuralgia: Simple technique for a complex disease. Journal of Clinical and Diagnostic Research. 2016;**10**(3):ZJ05-ZJ06

[12] Zhang H, Lian Y, Ma Y, Chen Y, He C, Xie N, et al. Two doses of botulinum toxin type A for the treatment of trigeminal neuralgia: Observation of therapeutic effect from a randomized, double-blind, placebo-controlled trial. The Journal of Headache and Pain. 2014;**15**:65

[13] Zakrzewska JM, Nally FF, Flint SR. Cryotherapy in the management of paroxysmal trigeminal neuralgia. Four year follow up of 39 patients. Journal of Maxillofacial Surgery. 1986;**14**(1):5-7

[14] Ali FM, Prasant M, Pai D, Aher VA, Kar S, Safiya T. Peripheral neurectomies: A treatment option for trigeminal neuralgia in rural practice. Journal of Neurosciences in Rural Practice. 2012;**3**(2):152-157

[15] Allam N, Brasil-Neto JP, Brown G, Tomaz C. Injections of botulinum toxin type a produce pain alleviation in intractable trigeminal neuralgia. The Clinical Journal of Pain. 2005;**21**(2):182-184

[16] Juniper RP. Trigeminal neuralgia—Treatment of the third division by radiologically controlled cryoblockade of the inferior dental nerve at the mandibular lingula: A study of 31 cases. British Journal of Oral and Maxillofacial Surgery. 1991;**29**(3):154-158

[17] Gronseth G, Cruccu G, Alksne J, Argoff C, Brainin M, Burchiel K, et al. Practice parameter: The diagnostic

evaluation and treatment of trigeminal neuralgia (an evidence-based review): Report of the Quality Standards Subcommittee of the American Academy of Neurology and the European Federation of Neurological Societies. Neurology. 2008;**71**(15):1183-1190

[18] Vasappa CK, Kapur S, Krovvidi H. Trigeminal neuralgia. BJA Education. 2016;**16**(10):353-356

[19] Farag E, Mounir-Soliman L. Brown's Atlas of Regional Anesthesia. Philadelphia: Elsevier; 2016

[20] Waldman SD. Atlas of Interventional Pain Management E-Book. Philadelphia: Elsevier—Health Sciences Division; 2014

[21] Gulur P, Wainger BJ, Young A. Head and Facial Trigeminal Neuralgia. Pain procedures in clinical practice. 2011. 297-304.

[22] McClenahan MF, Hillegass MG. Trigeminal nerve block. In: Yong RJ, Nguyen M, Nelson E, Urman RD, editors. Pain Medicine: An Essential Review. Cham: Springer International Publishing; 2017. pp. 275-277

[23] Peters JG, Nurmikko JT. Peripheral and gasserian ganglion-level procedures for the treatment of trigeminal neuralgia. The Clinical Journal of Pain. 2002;**18**(1):28-34

[24] Bick SKB, Eskandar EN. Surgical treatment of trigeminal neuralgia. Neurosurgery Clinics of North America. 2017;**28**(3):429-438

[25] Zakrzewska JM, Jassim S, Bulman JS. A prospective, longitudinal study on patients with trigeminal neuralgia who underwent radiofrequency thermocoagulation of the gasserian ganglion. Pain. 1999;**79**(1):51-58

[26] Nurmikko TJ, Eldridge PR. Trigeminal neuralgia—Pathophysiology, diagnosis and current treatment. British Journal of Anaesthesia. 2001;**87**(1):117-132

[27] Ammori MB, King AT, Siripurapu R, Herwadkar AV, Rutherford SA. Factors influencing decision-making and outcome in the surgical management of trigeminal neuralgia. Journal of Neurological Surgery. Part B, Skull Base. 2013;**74**(2):75-81

[28] Chang EF, Cheng JS, Lim DA, Barbaro NM. A review of percutaneous treatments for trigeminal neuralgia. Operative Neurosurgery. 2013;**10**(1):25-33

[29] Chen JF, Tu PH, Lee ST. Repeated percutaneous balloon compression for recurrent trigeminal neuralgia: A long-term study. World Neurosurgery. 2012;**77**(2):352-356

[30] Mullan S, Lichtor T. Percutaneous microcompression of the trigeminal ganglion for trigeminal neuralgia. Journal of Neurosurgery. 1983;**59**(6):1007-1012

[31] Hodaie M, Coello AF. Advances in the management of trigeminal neuralgia. Journal of Neurosurgical Sciences. 2013;**57**(1):13-21

[32] Aubuchon AC, Chan MD, Lovato JF, Balamucki CJ, Ellis TL, Tatter SB, et al. Repeat gamma knife radiosurgery for trigeminal neuralgia. International Journal of Radiation Oncology, Biology, Physics. 2011;**81**(4):1059-1065

[33] Kondziolka D, Zorro O, Lobato-Polo J, Kano H, Flannery TJ, Flickinger JC, et al. Gamma Knife stereotactic radiosurgery for idiopathic trigeminal neuralgia. Journal of Neurosurgery. 2010;**112**(4):758-765

[34] van Kleef M, van Genderen WE, Narouze S, Nurmikko TJ, van Zundert J,

Geurts JW, et al. Trigeminal neuralgia. Pain Practice. 2009;**9**(4):252-259

[35] Hitotsumatsu T, Matsushima T, Inoue T. Microvascular decompression for treatment of trigeminal neuralgia, hemifacial spasm, and glossopharyngeal neuralgia: Three surgical approach variations: Technical note. Neurosurgery. 2003;**53**(6):1436-1441. Discussion 42-3

[36] Rhoton AL Jr. The cerebellopontine angle and posterior fossa cranial nerves by the retrosigmoid approach. Neurosurgery. 2000;**47** (3 Suppl):S93-S129

[37] Matsushima T, Yamaguchi T, Inoue TK, Matsukado K, Fukui M. Recurrent trigeminal neuralgia after microvascular decompression using an interposing technique. Teflon felt adhesion and the sling retraction technique. Acta Neurochirurgica. 2000;**142**(5):557-561

[38] Jin HS, Shin JY, Kim YC, Lee SC, Choi EJ, Lee PB, et al. Predictive factors associated with success and failure for radiofrequency thermocoagulation in patients with trigeminal neuralgia. Pain Physician. 2015;**18**(6):537-545

[39] Berk C, Kanpolat Y, Savas A, Bekar A. Percutaneous controlled radiofrequency trigeminal rhizotomy for the treatment of idiopathic trigeminal neuralgia: 25-year experience with 1600 patients. Neurosurgery. 2001;**48**(3):524-534

[40] Noorani I, Lodge A, Vajramani G, Sparrow O. Comparing percutaneous treatments of trigeminal neuralgia: 19 years of experience in a single centre. Stereotactic and Functional Neurosurgery. 2016;**94**(2):75-85

[41] Guidetti B, Fraioli B, Cruccu G, Manfredi M, Esposito V. Treatment of trigeminal neuralgia by thermocoagulation, glycerolization, and percutaneous compression of the gasserian ganglion and/or retrogasserian rootlets: Long-term results and therapeutic protocol. Neurosurgery. 1989;**24**(2):239-245

[42] Blomstedt PC, Bergenheim AT. Technical difficulties and perioperative complications of retrogasserian glycerol rhizotomy for trigeminal neuralgia. Stereotactic and Functional Neurosurgery. 2002;**79**(3-4):168-181

[43] Lobato RD, Rivas JJ, Sarabia R, Lamas E. Percutaneous microcompression of the gasserian ganglion for trigeminal neuralgia. Journal of Neurosurgery. 1990;**72**(4):546-553

[44] de Siqueira SR, da Nobrega JC, de Siqueira JT, Teixeira MJ. Frequency of postoperative complications after balloon compression for idiopathic trigeminal neuralgia: Prospective study. Oral Surgery, Oral Medicine, Oral Pathology, Oral Radiology, and Endodontics. 2006;**102**(5):e39-e45

[45] Broggi G, Ferroli P, Franzini A, Servello D, Dones I. Microvascular decompression for trigeminal neuralgia: Comments on a series of 250 cases, including 10 patients with multiple sclerosis. Journal of Neurology, Neurosurgery, and Psychiatry. 2000;**68**(1):59-64

[46] Barker FG 2nd, Jannetta PJ, Babu RP, Pomonis S, Bissonette DJ, Jho HD. Long-term outcome after operation for trigeminal neuralgia in patients with posterior fossa tumors. Journal of Neurosurgery. 1996;**84**(5):818-825

[47] Pollock BE, Stien KJ. Posterior fossa exploration for trigeminal neuralgia patients older than 70 years of age. Neurosurgery. 2011;**69**(6): 1255-1259, 9-60

[48] Barker FG 2nd, Jannetta PJ, Bissonette DJ, Larkins MV, Jho HD. The

long-term outcome of microvascular decompression for trigeminal neuralgia. The New England Journal of Medicine. 1996;**334**(17):1077-1083

[49] Zhu S, Rong Q, Chen S, Li X. Pterygopalatine fossa segment neurectomy of maxillary nerve through maxillary sinus route in treating trigeminal neuralgia. Journal of Cranio-Maxillo-Facial Surgery. 2013;**41**(7):652-656

[50] Freemont AJ, Millac P. The place of peripheral neurectomy in the management of trigeminal neuralgia. Postgraduate Medical Journal. 1981;**57**(664):75-76

[51] Oturai AB, Jensen K, Eriksen J, Madsen F. Neurosurgery for trigeminal neuralgia: Comparison of alcohol block, neurectomy, and radiofrequency coagulation. The Clinical Journal of Pain. 1996;**12**(4):311-315

[52] Murali R, Rovit RL. Are peripheral neurectomies of value in the treatment of trigeminal neuralgia? An analysis of new cases and cases involving previous radiofrequency gasserian thermocoagulation. Journal of Neurosurgery. 1996;**85**(3):435-437

[53] Piovesan EJ, Teive HG, Kowacs PA, Della Coletta MV, Werneck LC, Silberstein SD. An open study of botulinum-A toxin treatment of trigeminal neuralgia. Neurology. 2005;**65**(8):1306-1308

[54] Turk U, Ilhan S, Alp R, Sur H. Botulinum toxin and intractable trigeminal neuralgia. Clinical Neuropharmacology. 2005;**28**(4):161-162

[55] Ngeow WC, Nair R. Injection of botulinum toxin type A (BOTOX) into trigger zone of trigeminal neuralgia as a means to control pain. Oral Surgery, Oral Medicine, Oral Pathology, Oral Radiology, and Endodontics. 2010;**109**(3):e47-e50

[56] Zakrzewska JM. Cryotherapy for trigeminal neuralgia: A 10 year audit. The British Journal of Oral and Maxillofacial Surgery. 1991;**29**(1):1-4

[57] Zakrzewska JM. Cryotherapy in the management of paroxysmal trigeminal neuralgia. Journal of Neurology, Neurosurgery, and Psychiatry. 1987;**50**(4):485-487

[58] Zakrzewska JM, Nally FF. The role of cryotherapy (cryoanalgesia) in the management of paroxysmal trigeminal neuralgia: A six year experience. The British Journal of Oral and Maxillofacial Surgery. 1988;**26**(1):18-25

[59] Nurmikko TJ, Eldridge PR. Trigeminal neuralgia - pathophysiology, diagnosis and current treatment. British Journal of Anaesthesia. 2001;**87**(1):117-132